THE SILENT STRUGGLE

Rewiring Male Anxiety in a Modern World — Tools for Emotional Resilience in Work, Relationships, and Life

Rupin Joshi

Copyright © 2025 by Rupin Joshi

All rights reserved.

No portion of this book may be copied, stored in a retrieval system, or shared in any form—electronic, mechanical, photocopying, recording, or otherwise—without prior written permission from the publisher, except as permitted by applicable copyright law.

Disclaimer & Limitation of Liability

This book is intended for informational purposes only. The author and publisher make no representations or warranties regarding the accuracy, completeness, or applicability of the content provided. The strategies, insights, and recommendations shared herein are based on personal and professional experience but may not be suitable for every individual.

This book does not substitute for medical, psychological, or professional advice. Readers experiencing severe anxiety, distress, or mental health concerns are encouraged to seek the guidance of a qualified healthcare provider. Neither the author nor the publisher shall be liable for any loss, damage, or adverse consequences arising from the use of the information in this book.

The mention of any specific organizations, websites, or external resources is for informational purposes only and does not imply endorsement. Additionally, online resources referenced in this book may change over time and should be verified independently.

Trademarks

All trademarks mentioned in this book belong to their respective owners. Their inclusion does not imply endorsement or affiliation with the author or publisher.

Publishing Information

Author: Rupin Joshi   Editor: Seema

ISBN : 9789334258202

Self-Published

Dedication

To the men who wake up every day carrying a weight no one else can see,

who push forward despite the storms raging within. To those who have fought tirelessly against anxiety and depression, who have battled in silence, unseen and unheard. And to those we have lost—the brothers, the fathers, the sons, the friends.

One of them was a man I knew well, a man who gave so much to others but couldn't find the light for himself. His absence is felt in every unspoken word, in every moment he should have been here to witness.

This book is for you. For all of you.

May we break the silence, lift the weight, and stand together—so no man fights alone.

CONTENTS

CONTENTS 5

INTRODUCTION 8

CHAPTER 1: HOW ANXIETY MANIFESTS DIFFERENTLY IN MEN 15

CHAPTER 2: THE MODERN TRAPS 20

CHAPTER 3: REWIRING THE MALE BRAIN 32

CHAPTER 4: THE ART OF VULNERABILITY 37

CHAPTER 5: WORK WITHOUT BURNOUT 48

CHAPTER 6: RELATIONSHIPS THAT DON'T DRAIN YOU 53

CHAPTER 7: THE INVISIBLE LOAD OF FATHERHOOD 61

CHAPTER 8: CRAFTING A PERSONALIZED RESILIENCE TOOLKIT 72

CHAPTER 9: BROTHERHOOD AND COMMUNITY 79

CHAPTER 10: LEGACY OF STRENGTH—REDEFINING MASCULINITY FOR THE NEXT GENERATION 85

CHAPTER 11: BIOLOGY OF ANXIETY 101

COMPREHENSIVE ACTIONABLE STEPS TO MANAGE ANXIETY & STRESS 107

CRISIS HOTLINES: IMMEDIATE SUPPORT WHEN YOU NEED IT 112

SELF-ASSESSMENT CHECKLIST 113

AUTHOR'S NOTE: A FINAL WORD 115

INTRODUCTION

Let me start with a confession: I used to be part of the problem.

For over a decade, I thrived in the high-stakes world of tech—a realm where "success" meant 80-hour weeks, relentless investor pitches, and wearing stress like a badge of honour. As a software engineer turned executive, I built teams, shipped products, and chased promotions, all while numbing my anxiety with caffeine and the hollow rush of achievement. I called it "hustle." My body called it self-destruction.

It wasn't until I collapsed during a boardroom presentation—my vision blurring, hands trembling—that I realized the cost of the lies we tell men:

"Push through it."

"Real men don't cry."

"Weakness is failure."

That panic attack wasn't just a wake-up call. It was a revolution. I left my tech career, retrained as a psychotherapist, and dedicated my life to dismantling the toxic myths I'd once embodied.

Today, as a licensed therapist specializing in men's mental health, I blend hard-won corporate survival skills with clinical expertise. My clients aren't lab subjects—they're CEOs, veterans, stay-at-home dads, and everyone in between, all wrestling with the same question: How do I be strong without losing myself?

This book is my answer.

Men are struggling with anxiety and depression at rates we've never seen before. And yet, most suffer in silence. Some push through each day, carrying the weight alone. Others—far too many—don't make it through.

The statistics tell a brutal truth.

- In the U.S., nearly four out of five suicides are men. That's not a coincidence. (CDC, 2023)
- Suicide is the second leading cause of death for men under 45—more than car accidents, heart disease, or cancer.
- Globally, men are significantly less likely to seek therapy than women, even when they're in distress.
- In high-stress jobs, men are twice as likely to develop anxiety disorders, but they're also less likely to take time off for mental health.

And yet, despite these numbers, the conversation around men's mental health is still filled with stigma, shame, and silence.

The Male Anxiety Epidemic

Let's name the crisis:

- 1 in 5 men will experience anxiety in their lifetime—but less than 30% seek help (APA, 2023).
- Male suicide rates are 3.7x higher than women's, with middle-aged men most at risk (CDC, 2022).
- Post-pandemic, workplace burnout among men surged 42%, yet 65% still hide symptoms to avoid being seen as "unreliable" (Gallup, 2023).

<u>Anxiety in men isn't a personal failing</u>—it's a cultural one. We've been handed a script that equates masculinity with emotional suppression, self-reliance, and endless stoicism. But here's what I've learned in my own struggle: The strongest men aren't those who hide their struggles—they're the ones who face them.

Why Men Stay Silent?

In my work with CEOs, veterans, stay-at-home dads, and everyone in between, I've seen three toxic myths keep men trapped:

1. The Myth of Weakness: "Asking for help means I'm broken."

Reality: Vulnerability is the foundation of courage. It takes far more strength to say "I'm not okay" than to bury pain.

2. The Myth of Burden: "My problems will overwhelm others."

Reality: Your loved ones want to support you—but they can't if you don't let them in.

3. The Myth of Invincibility: "I should handle this alone."

Reality: Humans are wired for connection. Even lions rely on their pride.

Post-Pandemic World & Male Anxiety

The pandemic didn't just change how we work or socialize—it reshaped the mental health landscape, especially for men. As we adapt to a world where Zoom calls replace watercooler chats and LinkedIn profiles feel as curated as Instagram feeds, men are grappling with silent stressors: endless screen time, shrinking social circles, questionable eating habits, and the relentless pressure to "keep up" in a tech-driven job market. Let's unpack these layers.

1. Social Media & Screen Time: The Double-Edged Sword

Post-pandemic, screen time isn't just about Netflix binges. Men now spend 4+ hours daily on social media (Pew Research, 2022), up 35% from pre-2020. While platforms promise connection, studies reveal a darker side:

- Men logging >3 hours/day on apps like Instagram or Twitter are 30% more likely to report depression (Journal of Affective Disorders, 2021).

- Constant exposure to "successful" peers fuels comparison anxiety. One survey found 42% of men feel inadequate about career progress after scrolling LinkedIn (APA, 2023).

And it's not just mental strain—blue light from screens disrupts sleep, a critical factor for mood. Men with poor sleep are 2x as likely to develop anxiety (CDC, 2022).

2. The Loneliness Epidemic: Missing the "Third Place"

For many men, pre-pandemic socializing happened organically—gyms, sports bars, or office lunches. Post-COVID, 40% of men report having fewer close friends (Survey Centre on American Life, 2023). This isolation hits hard:

- Men with weak social ties are 25% more likely to die prematurely (Harvard Study, 2020), and loneliness correlates with higher cortisol levels, worsening stress.

- Remote work exacerbates this; 1 in 3 remote workers (mostly men in tech/IT roles) say they've lost work friendships (Gallup, 2022).

3. Nutrition: The Overlooked Mental Health Catalyst

Lockdowns turned fridges into 24/7 cafeterias, but convenience often trumped health. Men's diets shifted toward processed foods, with 35% eating fewer veggies post-pandemic (NIH, 2023). Poor nutrition isn't just a physical risk:

- Diets high in sugar/fat are linked to a 28% increase in depressive symptoms in men (British Journal of Nutrition, 2022).

- Deficiencies in magnesium and vitamin D—common in male diets—worsen anxiety (Mayo Clinic, 2021).

4. The Tech Treadmill: "Upskilling or Obsolete?"

Tech innovation isn't slowing down, and neither is the pressure to adapt. Men in fields like IT, engineering, and finance report:

- 60% feel "constant pressure" to learn new skills (LinkedIn, 2023)—think AI tools, coding bootcamps, or ChatGPT.
- 45% tie their self-worth to job relevance (Gallup, 2023), leading to burnout. One DevOps engineer shared, "I spend weekends studying cloud certifications. It's exhausting, but I can't risk falling behind."

Let me share a story with you at this point, which I believe represents a genuine case of what I see as a growing problem, John, a 38-year-old father of two, used to work as a machine operator at a manufacturing plant in the Midwest. For over a decade, he took pride in his job, providing for his family and feeling a sense of purpose. But in 2018, the plant introduced automated machinery, and John was laid off. Despite his experience, he struggled to find stable work in a job market increasingly dominated by tech-driven roles.

To make ends meet, John started driving for a ride-sharing app. The gig was flexible, but the long hours and lack of benefits left him exhausted and anxious. He missed the camaraderie of his old workplace and felt isolated in his car, scrolling through social media during downtime. Online, he saw former colleagues thriving in new careers or friends boasting about promotions, which made him question his own worth.

At home, John felt the pressure to be the "rock" for his family. His wife had taken on a part-time job, and while he appreciated her support, it challenged his identity as the primary provider. He didn't want to burden her with his worries, so he bottled up his stress, turning to late-night TV and video games to cope. His sleep suffered, and he started feeling irritable and disconnected from his kids.

One evening, after a particularly gruelling day, John found himself sitting in his car, staring at his phone. He felt a deep sense of loneliness, even though he was surrounded by people—both online and in his community. He thought about reaching out to an old friend or seeking help, but the fear of being judged or seen as weak stopped him.

"Men don't talk about this stuff," he told himself.

John's story is not unique. It reflects the struggles of millions of men navigating a rapidly changing world where traditional roles are disappearing, economic pressures are mounting, and societal expectations remain rigid. The combination of job insecurity, social isolation, and the stigma around mental health creates a perfect storm for mental health challenges.

Part 1: Understanding Anxiety in a Man's World

CHAPTER 1: HOW ANXIETY MANIFESTS DIFFERENTLY IN MEN

The Day I Punched a Wall (And What It Taught Me)

Let's rewind to my tech days. I was 32, leading a team of 50 engineers, and had just blown a presentation to investors. Instead of admitting I was drowning in stress, I channelled my inner Hulk. On the drive home, I white-knuckled the steering wheel, yelled at a guy who cut me off, and later—after my kids were asleep—slammed my fist into the drywall of my garage.

When my wife found me icing my hand, she didn't ask, "Are you okay?" She said, "You're scaring me."

That moment wasn't just about a bruised ego (or a bruised fist). It was a crash course in how men misinterpret anxiety as anger—and how our bodies often scream what our minds won't say.

Physical Symptoms: When Anxiety Wears a Mask

For men, anxiety rarely shows up as trembling hands or tearful breakdowns. It's more like a wolf in wolf's clothing—disguised as:

Anger: Road rage, snapping at colleagues, or simmering resentment over minor slights.

Irritability: That "Why is everyone so damn annoying?" feeling during a packed commute.

Restlessness: Pacing, nail-biting, or obsessively checking emails at 2 a.m.

Why?

Biologically, men are wired to externalize stress. Testosterone, our "action hormone," primes us to respond to threats with aggression or dominance—a leftover from when "anxiety" meant "sabre-toothed tiger nearby." But in modern life, there's no tiger. Just traffic, deadlines, and passive-aggressive Slack messages.

Case Study: The CEO Who Couldn't Sit Still

One client—a founder you've probably used an app from—came to me insisting he had "ADHD." Turns out, his constant fidgeting and outbursts at meetings weren't a focus issue. They were his body's way of screaming, *"I'm terrified this company will fail, and I'll lose everything."*

We didn't start with meditation. We started with push-ups.

Science Byte:

- Testosterone surges during stress can heighten aggression (hence the wall-punching).
- Cortisol (the "stress hormone") stays elevated longer in men than women, keeping us locked in fight-or-flight mode—even when the "threat" is just an overflowing inbox.

Emotional Symptoms: The Sadness We Swallow

Here's the paradox: Men do feel sadness, fear, and shame. We just Armor up instead of admitting it.

I'll never forget a client—a retired Marine—who sat stone-faced in my office for weeks. Then one day, he whispered, *"I cried in my truck after dropping my daughter at college. I didn't even go to her graduation. I was... scared."*

For men, sadness often morphs into:

- **Numbness:** The "I don't feel anything" lie we tell ourselves.
- **Isolation:** Cancelling plans, zoning out during family dinners.
- **Self-Blame:** "I'm failing as a husband/father/provider."

Why Men Mislabel Emotions

Growing up, boys get two messages:

1. "Don't be a sissy."
2. "Fix it or shut up about it."

Result? We treat emotions like a programming bug—something to troubleshoot alone. But anxiety isn't a glitch. It's a signal.

Example:

- **Physical:** Clenched jaw during your kid's recital = *"I'm anxious I'm not present enough."*
- **Emotional:** Avoiding friends after a layoff = *"I'm ashamed I can't provide."*

Testosterone & Cortisol: The Hormonal Tango

Let's geek out on biochemistry—without the jargon.

1. **Testosterone:**

The Good: Fuels confidence, focus, and sexual health.

The Bad: High levels can make us overreact to stress (think: arguing with a barista over a wrong order).

The Fix: Channel it physically. Lift weights, sprint, chop wood—anything that lets your body "fight" stress constructively.

2. **Cortisol:**

The Good: Sharpens focus in short bursts (e.g., nailing a presentation).

The Bad: Chronic stress = cortisol on overdrive. This shuts down "non-essential" systems (like digestion, sleep, empathy).

The Fix: Burn it off. A 10-minute walk after work tells your body, "The threat's gone. Stand down."

A Personal Hack: The 90-Second Rule

When cortisol hijacks your brain:

Notice: "My chest is tight. Cortisol's spiking."

Move: Stand up. Stretch. Splash cold water on your face.

Redirect: Ask, "What's the real threat here?"

(*Spoiler: It's rarely the actual situation.*)

This isn't woo-woo. It's neurobiology.

Cortisol floods your system for 90 seconds—after that, it's your choice to keep revving.

Your Body Isn't Broken—It's Trying to Talk to You

Years ago, I treated a mechanic who came in for "anger issues." During sessions, he'd tap his boot nervously. One day, I asked, "What's your body saying right now?"

He froze. Then admitted, *"I'm... scared my wife's going to leave me. I don't know how to be vulnerable."*

His tapping foot wasn't anger. It was fear in work boots.

Key Takeaways:

- Anger ≠ You: It's often anxiety in a Halloween costume.
- Cortisol is a crappy long-term fuel: Burn it, don't let it burn you.
- Sadness isn't weakness: It's data. Get curious, not judgmental.

Try This Tonight-

For Physical Symptoms: Do 10 push-ups the second you feel rage bubbling. It's not about fitness—it's about giving testosterone a job.

For Emotional Numbness: Write one sentence starting with "I'm afraid..." Then burn it. No one has to see it.

CHAPTER 2: THE MODERN TRAPS

The Night I Became a Keyboard Warrior

Let's rewind to 2021. I was scrolling through LinkedIn at midnight, bleary-eyed, when I saw a post from an old tech colleague: *"Just closed a $10M funding round! #HustleHarder."* My gut twisted. I'd just spent the day consoling a suicidal client, forgotten my son's soccer game, and eaten cold pizza over the sink. In a fit of shame, I fired off a passive-aggressive comment: *"Must be nice to have time for self-promotion."*

The next morning, I deleted it—but the shame lingered. That's when I realized: *Modern life isn't just stressful for men. It's rigged to exploit our deepest insecurities.*

Trap 1: Social Media Comparison—The Dopamine Deception

Story: Meet "Alex," a 34-year-old engineer who came to me with crippling imposter syndrome. His trigger? Instagram. He'd scroll through influencers' "perfect" lives—six-pack abs, luxury cars, #Blessed captions—and seethe. *"I work 60 hours a week and still feel like a loser,"* he admitted.

The Science: Social media hijacks our primal need for status. Every like trigger dopamine (the "winning the hunt" chemical), but men's brains also flood with cortisol when comparing ourselves to others.

Status Anxiety: We're hardwired to measure ourselves against the tribe. But Instagram isn't a tribe—it's a global stage of highlight reels.

The Fix:

- **Unfollow *"Motivation"*:** If an account makes you feel less than, mute it. Your mental health isn't worth the "hustle porn."

- **Compare Up, Not Down:** Instead of *"Why isn't that me?"* ask *"What part of their journey am I not seeing?"* (Spoiler: Debt, divorce, burnout.)

Trap 2: Financial Pressure—The Provider Paradox

Story: "James," a laid-off oil rig worker, told me through gritted teeth, *"I'd rather die than let my family see me fail."* He'd been sleeping in his truck for weeks, too ashamed to go home.

The Science: Financial stress activates the survival brain—the same region that lights up during physical threats. For men, whose self-worth is often tied to providing, this becomes a 24/7 cortisol drip.

The Data: Men are 3x more likely to cite money as their top stressor than women (APA, 2023).

The Fix:

- **Reframe "Provider":** Your value isn't your pay check. It's your presence. (Yes, even if TikTok dads make artisan sourdough look easy.)

- **The 3-Minute Budget:** Write one financial fear and one action step. Example: *"Fear: Losing the house. Step: Call the mortgage company TODAY."*

Trap 3: Remote Work Isolation—The Zoom Zombie Effect

Story: During lockdown, a software developer named "Mark" started having panic attacks. His only human interaction? Slack emojis and his cat's judgmental stares. "I miss the guys," he said. "Even Bob from Accounting."

The Science: Men bond through side-by-side interaction (think sports, work banter). Remote work strips this away, spiking loneliness—a bigger health risk than smoking (CDC, 2022).

The Testosterone Twist: Low social connection reduces testosterone, fuelling lethargy and depression.

The Fix:

- **Create a "Third Place":** Join a garage gym, trivia night, or Dungeons & Dragons group. No, it's not "cringe"—it's survival.

- **Virtual Watercoolers:** Schedule a 10-minute video call with a coworker just to bitch about the Wi-Fi. No agenda.

Trap 4: "Always On" Culture—Burnout's Breeding Ground

Story: In my tech days, I wore sleeplessness like a medal. Then, at 3 a.m. one Tuesday, I hallucinated my spreadsheet was talking to me. My boss's response?

"Take a nap and get back to it."

The Science: Chronic stress shrinks the prefrontal cortex (your decision-making hub) and enlarges the amygdala (your panic button). Translation: Burnout makes you dumber and more reactive.

The Male Toll: Men are 40% less likely to take mental health days, fearing career repercussions (Harvard Business Review, 2023).

The Fix:

- **The 8-8-8 Rule:** 8 hours work, 8 hours rest, 8 hours whatever the hell you want. Guard those buckets fiercely.

- **Email Graveyard:** Turn off notifications after 6 p.m. If the company burns down without you, they'll call.

Your Escape Plan

Audit Your Inputs: Ditch apps that sell insecurity. Follow accounts that make you feel enough.

Talk Money Early: Normalize financial chats with your partner before the 3 a.m. cold sweats.

Touch Grass (Literally): Grounding your bare feet on soil reduces cortisol. Science says so.

Key Takeaways:

- Social media is a casino—you always lose when playing someone else's game.
- Financial fear shrinks under sunlight. Shame grows in darkness.
- Isolation is a slow killer. Connection is a lifeline—even if it's awkward at first.

Anxiety & Depression Assessment for Men:

"The Mirror Test"

A dual-purpose tool to quantify symptoms + uncover emotional patterns

"You've mapped your mind's maze in the game. Now, let's hold up a mirror. This isn't about labels or judgment—it's about seeing patterns, like noticing cracks in armour so you can mend them. The questions ahead are designed to meet you where you are: blunt, practical, and free of therapy-speak. Your answers will translate into a snapshot of your mental 'weather'—and a compass for what to work on. No right or wrong. Just honesty. Ready to turn fog into focus?"

Structure of the Test

15 questions (5 per category: Stress, Anxiety, Depression) using a 0–3 scale:

0 = Never | 1 = Rarely | 2 = Often | 3 = Always

Part 1: Symptom Measurement

The Questionnaire

(Answer Each Question using 0-3 scale, put score inside box)

Stress (S)

1. I feel irritable over small things, like traffic or minor mistakes. ☐

2. My muscles feel tense (jaw, shoulders, back) even when resting. ☐

3. I use alcohol, gaming, or binge-watching to "zone out." ☐

4. I struggle to fall asleep because my mind races about tomorrow. ☐

5. I feel guilty when I'm not being productive. ☐

The Silent Struggle

(Answer Each Question using 0-3 scale, put score inside box)

Anxiety (A)

1. I replay past conversations, worried I sounded awkward.

2. My chest feels tight or my heart races for no clear reason.

3. I avoid social plans because I might "run out of things to say."

4. I overprepare for tasks to avoid criticism (e.g., triple-checking emails).

5. I imagine worst-case scenarios about my job/relationships.

(Answer Each Question using 0-3 scale, put score inside box)

Depression (D)

1. I feel emotionally numb, even with people I care about. ☐

2. Hobbies I used to love (sports, gaming, etc.) feel pointless now. ☐

3. I criticize myself harshly ("I'm failing" or "I'm weak"). ☐

4. My appetite has drastically increased/decreased without trying. ☐

5. I feel like a burden to others when I share my struggles. ☐

Scoring Criteria: How to Measure Your Stress, Anxiety, and Depression Levels

(It's like a "weather report" for your mind!)

Add Up Your Scores:

Stress (Add your answers to questions under stress Questionnaire)

STRESS SCORE =

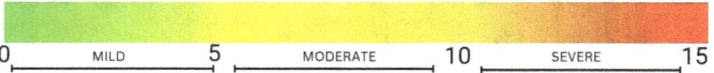

Anxiety (Add your answers to questions under Anxiety Questionnaire)

ANXIETY SCORE =

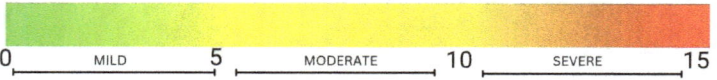

Depression (Add your answers to questions under Depression Questionnaire)

DEPRESSION SCORE =

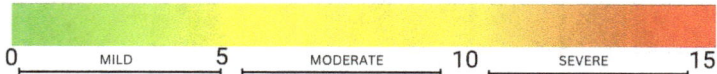

Part 2: Personality Reflection: What Your Answers Say About You

(Think of this as your "coping style cheat sheet.")

Your answers reveal how you handle tough emotions. Look at which category (Stress, Anxiety, Depression) has your highest score(s). Then match it to one of these four profiles:

Profile 1: The Pressure-Cooker Protector

Signs: **High Stress + Anxiety scores.**

You're the "fixer" who bottles up emotions to avoid burdening others.

What to Work On:

- Say "no" to one extra task this week.
- Try "rage cardio" (sprints, punching a pillow) to release tension.

Profile 2: The Silent Strategist

Signs: **High Anxiety + Depression scores.**

You overthink to avoid feeling vulnerable ("If I plan everything, I won't fail").

What to Work On:

- Share one small worry with a friend (e.g., "Work's been hectic").
- Write down 3 things you can't control (let them go like a balloon).

Profile 3: The High-Octane Achiever

Signs: **High Stress + Depression scores.**

Your self-worth is tied to achievements ("If I stop, I'm worthless").

What to Work On:

- Redefine rest as "productive" (e.g., "Rest = recharging my focus").
- Do a hobby badly (e.g., doodle stick figures) to break perfectionism.

Profile 4: The Isolated Innovator

Signs: **All three scores are moderately high.**

You withdraw when stressed ("I'll handle it alone"), which deepens loneliness.

What to Work On:

- Join a low-pressure group (e.g., a hiking club, gaming Discord).
- Text a friend a meme—no need for deep talks.

Part 2: Building Emotional Resilience

CHAPTER 3: REWIRING THE MALE BRAIN

The Day I Jumped into a Frozen Lake (And Didn't Die)

Let me paint you a scene: New Zealand, 2015. I'm standing on the edge of Lake Wakatipu, snow crunching under my boots, wearing nothing but swim trunks and a death wish. My Kiwi buddies dared me to take the plunge—"For mental toughness, mate!"—and my inner tech-bro ego couldn't refuse.

Three seconds underwater felt like three lifetimes. But when I surfaced, gasping and alive, something clicked: Extreme cold doesn't just shock the body—it reboots the brain.

This chapter isn't about becoming an ice-swimming masochist. It's about hacking your biology to turn anxiety into armour.

Tool 1: Cold Exposure—The Stress Vaccine

Science Simplified:

- Cold showers/ice baths trigger acute stress, activating your sympathetic nervous system (the "fight-or-flight" response).

- Repeated exposure teaches your brain: "This discomfort won't kill me." Over time, daily stressors (traffic, deadlines) feel smaller in comparison.

Client Story:

"Tom," a firefighter with PTSD, started with 30-second cold showers. Within weeks, he reported: "Panic attacks dropped by half. Now when my alarm blares, I'm calm—like my body remembers it can handle chaos."

Your Starter Kit:

- End Your Shower on Cold: 30 seconds to start. Breathe through the gasp reflex.

- Scream if You Need To: It's science—vocalizing reduces perceived pain.

Why It Works for Men:

Cold exposure taps into our primal love of challenges. It's not self-care—it's a damn conquest.

Tool 2: Breathwork—The Stealth Weapon Against Panic

The Wim Hof Method (Minus the Cult Vibe):

- Step 1: Inhale deeply through the nose (4 seconds).

- Step 2: Exhale slowly through the mouth (6 seconds).

- Repeat for 5 minutes.

The Silent Struggle

Science Simplified:

Extending exhales activates the parasympathetic nervous system, lowering heart rate and cortisol. Men often reject "meditation" as too passive—but breathwork is active control.

Client Story:

"Raj," a Wall Street trader, used breathwork to survive boardroom panic attacks. "I'd mute Zoom and do the 4-6 breath. Now I outlast every prick in that room."

Pro Tip: Pair breathwork with a physical anchor (gripping a stress ball, stomping your feet) to engage the male brain's action bias.

Tool 3: Strength Training—Lifting Weights, Lowering Anxiety

More Than Gains:

- Strength training boosts testosterone (improving mood) and BDNF (a protein that repairs stress-damaged neurons).

- The ritual of progressive overload (lifting heavier each week) mirrors psychological resilience.

Client Story:

"Mike," a divorced dad, swapped nightly bourbon for deadlifts. "Now when I feel the rage coming, I hit the gym. Anger becomes energy, not explosions."

Your No-BS Routine:

3x Weekly: Squats, push-ups, pull-ups. No fancy equipment needed.

Track Progress: Men thrive on measurable wins. Write down every PR.

Why It's Not Just Exercise:

Lifting is embodied CBT—proof that incremental effort yields tangible results.

Tool 4: CBT as Mental Discipline—Reprogram Your Inner Drill Sergeant

CBT Reframed:

Cognitive Behavioural Therapy isn't about "positive vibes." It's mental martial arts—training your brain to counterpunch toxic thoughts.

The 3-Step Fight Plan:

1. Spot the Enemy: Identify distorted thoughts ("I'm a failure if I ask for help").

2. Interrogate the Evidence: "Would I call my buddy a failure for needing a hand?"

3. Launch a Counterstrike: Replace the lie with a mantra ("Strength is knowing my limits").

Client Story:

"Derek," an Army vet, used CBT to silence his inner critic after a career-ending injury. "I told myself, 'Adapting isn't surrender—it's strategy.' Now I coach other vets."

Metaphor for Men:

Think of CBT as a mental gym. You wouldn't skip leg day—why skip brain day?

The Synergy Effect: Stack Your Tools

Morning Routine for the Modern Man:

- 5:30 AM: Cold shower (90 seconds). Wake up the warrior.
- 5:35 AM: Breathwork (5 minutes). Calm the storm.
- 6:00 AM: Strength train (30 minutes). Forge discipline.
- Throughout the Day: CBT check-ins ("Is this thought useful or bullshit?").

Why Stacking Works:

Each tool reinforces the others. Cold exposure builds stress resilience, breathwork maintains clarity, strength training fuels confidence, and CBT keeps your mindset tactical.

Key Takeaways

- Cold Exposure: Teaches your body stress is survivable.
- Breathwork: Lets you hijack panic in real-time.
- Strength Training: Turns anxiety into actionable energy.
- CBT: Is the playbook for mental warfare.

CHAPTER 4: THE ART OF VULNERABILITY

The Email I Almost Didn't Send

In 2018, I sat in my office at 2 a.m., staring at a draft email to my wife. We'd been fighting for weeks—about money, parenting, my workaholism. My first instinct? Double down. Defend. Deny. But that night, I typed three words I'd never said aloud:

"I'm scared I'm failing you."

Sending it felt like jumping off a cliff. Her reply? "I'm scared too. Let's fix this."

Vulnerability didn't fix our marriage overnight. But it gave us a map instead of a minefield. This chapter isn't about crying. It's about strategic courage—using vulnerability as a tool to rebuild trust, intimacy, and respect.

Why Vulnerability Feels Like Kryptonite (And How to Rebrand It)

Myth: Vulnerability = weakness.

Truth: Vulnerability is precision-guided emotional risk-taking.

The Science of Connection:

Studies show men who practice vulnerability have 37% lower cortisol levels during conflicts (Journal of Personality, 2021). Oxytocin (the "bonding hormone") spikes during honest conversations, countering anxiety's isolation effect.

Testosterone's Role: Contrary to myth, vulnerability doesn't lower testosterone. In fact, men who embrace emotional honesty show healthier testosterone profiles by reducing chronic stress (Psychneuroendocrinology, 2022).

The Male Dilemma:

We're taught to equate vulnerability with loss of control. But as one client, a former MMA fighter, told me:

"You think I 'win' fights by clenching harder? Nah. I flow. Adapt. Let my guard down to strike smarter."

Cultural Barriers:

In collectivist cultures (e.g., Asian, Latino), vulnerability may clash with familial duty. A client, "Hiro," shared: "In Japan, admitting stress feels like betraying my family's sacrifice."

Reframe: Vulnerability as honouring your lineage by breaking cycles of silent suffering.

Case Studies: Vulnerability in Action

Case Study 1: The CEO Who Learned to Say "I Don't Know"

Background: "Mark," 45, founder of a tech unicorn, came to me after his wife threatened divorce. "She says I'm a robot. But if I'm vulnerable, my team will think I'm weak."

Breakthrough Moment: During a board meeting, Mark admitted, "I don't have the answer. Let's figure this out together." His team's response? Relief. One VP later confessed, "We thought you were hiding something."

Steps He Took:

- Start Small: He began sharing minor uncertainties at work ("I'm torn between these two strategies").

- Home Practice: Told his wife, "I'm scared I've prioritized work over us. Can we talk?"

Outcome: Promoted to Chairman (for fostering collaboration), saved his marriage.

Takeaway: Vulnerability isn't about dumping emotions—it's about inviting collaboration.

Case Study 2: The Veteran Who Reconnected with His Son

Background: "Carl," 52, ex-Marine, hadn't spoken to his 18-year-old son in two years. "He thinks I'm a heartless drill sergeant."

Breakthrough Moment: Carl wrote his son a letter:

"When you came out as gay, I froze. Not because I didn't accept you—because I was terrified of saying the wrong thing. I'm sorry. I want to learn."

Steps He Took:

- Use "I" Statements: "I felt scared," not "You made me scared."

- Ask Questions: "Can you help me understand what you need from me?"

Outcome: His son replied, "Dad, you trying is enough." They now attend Pride together.

Takeaway: Vulnerability bridges gaps when pride builds walls.

The Silent Struggle

Case Study 3: The Immigrant Father Who Broke the Silence

Background: "Ahmed," 60, a Pakistani-American taxi driver, hid his depression for years. "In my village, men don't cry. But my chest aches every night."

Breakthrough Moment: At a family dinner, Ahmed confessed: "I've been carrying a darkness. I need your help to lighten it." His sons, initially stunned, later pooled money for therapy.

Steps He Took:

- Leverage Metaphors: Framed emotions as a shared burden ("darkness") rather than a personal flaw.

- Cultural Bridge: Used communal values (family honour) to justify seeking help.

Takeaway: Vulnerability can respect tradition while rewriting its rules.

Scripts for Tough Conversations

Scenario 1: Telling Your Partner, You're Struggling

Old Script: "I'm fine. Just work stress." (Leads to resentment)

New Script: "I've been feeling overwhelmed lately, and I'm scared of letting you down. I need your support, but I'm not sure how to ask."

Why It Works: Names the emotion (scared), invites partnership (support), and admits uncertainty (not sure).

Scenario 2: Admitting a Mistake to Your Team

Old Script: "The delay wasn't my fault. The client changed specs." (Defensive)

New Script: "I underestimated this project's complexity, and that's on me. Let's regroup and fix this—I need your best ideas."

Why It Works: Takes ownership (on me), shifts to solutions (regroup), empowers others (your ideas).

Scenario 3: Apologizing to a Friend

Old Script: "Sorry if you were offended." (Passive-aggressive)

New Script: "I messed up. What I said was disrespectful, and I hate that I hurt you. How can I make this right?"

Why It Works: Specific (disrespectful), emotional accountability (hate), action-oriented (make it right).

Scenario 4: Talking to a Parent About Aging

Old Script: "You're fine. Stop worrying." (Dismissive)

New Script: "I'm scared about your health, and I don't want to face it alone. Can we make a plan together?"

Why It Works: Acknowledges mutual fear (scared), frames collaboration (plan together).

Scenario 5: Navigating Workplace Sexism

Old Script: "I don't see the problem." (Complicit)

New Script: "That comment didn't sit right with me. Can we discuss how to foster a more inclusive team?"

Why It Works: Moral clarity (didn't sit right), proactive resolution (inclusive team).

The Vulnerability Hangover: Surviving the Aftermath

Even successful vulnerability can leave men feeling raw. Here's how to cope:

Name the Shame: *"I feel exposed right now. That's normal."*

Ground Yourself:

Physical: Do 5 minutes of breathwork or lift weights.

Environmental: Walk barefoot on grass (earthing reduces cortisol).

Debrief: If the conversation went well, text a trusted friend: "Took a risk today. Proud of myself."

When It Backfires:

Example: "I told my brother I felt neglected, and he laughed."

Response: "His reaction says more about him than you. You still honoured your truth."

Client Hack: "Jake," a lawyer, keeps a "Courage Log" where he writes down every vulnerable moment. "Reading it reminds me I've survived 100% of my fears."

Vulnerability Across Cultures: A Global Playbook

Middle Eastern Men

Barrier: In many Arab cultures, vulnerability is seen as a threat to *sharaf* (family honour) or *ird* (dignity). Men often suppress emotions to avoid appearing "weak" in front of kin or community.

Strategy: Frame vulnerability as wisdom, not weakness. Example: "Honouring our family means addressing pain before it becomes a wound. Let's heal together."

South Asian Men (India, Pakistan, Bangladesh)

Barrier: The "provider" role in joint families' pressures men to suppress struggles. Mental health is often stigmatized as a "Western problem."

Strategy: Use communal language. Example: "Just as we care for our temple, we must care for our minds. Our family's strength depends on it."

Indigenous/Native American Men

Barrier: Historical trauma and colonial erasure have equated vulnerability with risk. Stoicism is valorised as survival.

Strategy: Reconnect with storytelling traditions. Example: "Our ancestors shared struggles around the fire. Let's carry their courage by speaking our truths."

Scandinavian Men (Sweden, Norway, Denmark)

Barrier: The Law of Jante ("Don't think you're special") discourages emotional expression to maintain social equality.

Strategy: Normalize vulnerability as collective care. Example: "By sharing our burdens, we strengthen the whole village. Your pain is ours too."

Nigerian Men

Barrier: Hypermasculine "Big Man" ideals prioritize dominance. Vulnerability is misread as incompetence.

Strategy: Link openness to leadership. Example: "A true leader knows when to lean on his tribe. Even the iroko tree bends in the storm."

Mediterranean Men (Greek, Italian)

Barrier: Passionate expression is accepted, but vulnerability (e.g., admitting insecurity) conflicts with machismo ideals.

Strategy: Tie emotions to legacy. Example: "Our nonnos wept when they rebuilt after the war. Strength is passing their resilience to our children."

Eastern European Men (Poland, Russia)

Barrier: Historical hardships bred stoicism; vulnerability is seen as a luxury or betrayal of resilience.

Strategy: Reframe vulnerability as strategic resilience. Example: "Our fathers survived wars by relying on comrades. We survive today by relying on each other."

Maori Men (New Zealand)

Barrier: Traditional *tane* (manhood) emphasizes physical strength and silent endurance.

Strategy: Use *whakawhanaungatanga* (relationship-building). Example: "In the wharenui (meeting house), we speak with hearts as well as fists."

Jewish Men

Barrier: The "Jewish mother" stereotype overshadows men's emotional needs, while historical persecution fuels a "never again" defensiveness.

Strategy: Leverage cultural humour and textual tradition. Example: "Even King David wrote psalms of doubt. It's Jewish to question—and to heal."

Caribbean Men

Barrier: Colonial legacies and "macho" tropes equate vulnerability with submissiveness.

Strategy: Celebrate communal resilience. Example: "Our islands survived hurricanes by standing together. Our hearts can too."

Q&A: Your Vulnerability Roadblocks

Q: "What if I'm rejected after being vulnerable?"

A: Rejection often reflects the other person's limitations, not your worth. As one client put it: "I'd rather be rejected for being real than loved for being fake."

Q: "How do I avoid oversharing?"

A: Vulnerability ≠ trauma dumping. Use the 30% Rule: Share 30% of what you're feeling initially, then gauge safety.

Q: "What if I cry?"

A: Tears are biological stress relievers. One study found men who cry during conflicts report higher relationship satisfaction (Emotion, 2020).

Exercises to Build Vulnerability Muscles

The Mirror Drill:

Stand in front of a mirror and say: "I'm feeling _____ today." Repeat until it feels less alien.

Gradual Exposure:

Week 1: Compliment a colleague sincerely.

Week 2: Admit a small mistake to your partner.

Week 3: Share a fear with a trusted friend.

Role-Play Rejection:

Practice scenarios with a therapist or friend. Example: "What if they laugh?" Prepares your nervous system for real-life risks.

Key Takeaways

- Vulnerability is a Skill: Start low-stakes (e.g., admitting a minor mistake) and build.
- Use Frameworks, Not Feelings: Scripts give structure when emotions overwhelm.
- It's Not About You: Vulnerability gives others permission to be human too.

Part 3: Anxiety in Key Life Domains

CHAPTER 5: WORK WITHOUT BURNOUT

The Day My AI Overlord Almost Broke Me

In 2023, I agreed to beta-test a productivity app that promised to "optimize every minute" of my life. By day three, it had scheduled my bathroom breaks, micromanaged my email replies, and sent my wife a calendar invite labelled "Discuss Relationship Efficiency." I lasted 72 hours before tossing my phone into a lake.

This chapter isn't just about surviving burnout—it's about reclaiming your humanity in an age where algorithms hijack your nervous system and ChatGPT writes your performance reviews. Let's dig into the modern traps and tools reshaping work, stress, and sanity.

1. Setting Boundaries in a Hustle-Culture World

The New Work Prison: Always On, Never Free

Digital Chains: Slack pings at midnight. Zoom fatigue. AI surveillance tools tracking keystrokes. The 9-to-5 is dead; now work is a 24/7 hostage situation.

Male Vulnerability: Men are 50% more likely to answer work emails after hours (Forbes, 2023), mistaking availability for ambition.

Science Bite:

Constant screen exposure reduces gray matter in the prefrontal cortex (your decision-making hub). Translation: Hustle culture makes you dumber. Blue light from devices suppresses melatonin, disrupting sleep cycles and spiking cortisol.

Case Study: The Dev Who Outsmarted His Algorithm

"Jake," a remote software engineer, used a script to auto-reply "I'm in deep work mode until 3 p.m." to all Slack messages. Productivity soared. His boss? Never noticed.

Boundary-Setting in the Age of AI

Step 1: Declare Digital Sovereignty

Tools:

- Freedom App: Block work apps post-6 p.m.

- Old-School Tactics: A $20 burner phone for weekends.

Script: "I'm offline after 7 p.m. to protect my focus. For emergencies, call twice—I'll assume someone's dying."

Step 2: Hack the Hustle Bots

AI Countermeasures:

- Use ChatGPT to draft "I'm at capacity" emails.

- Set OOO messages with teeth: "I'm hiking with my dog. Your email will self-destruct in 24 hours."

Step 3: The "Analog Hour" Ritual

No screens. No AI. Just pen, paper, and primal thinking.

Client Hack: A Silicon Valley exec sketches ideas on a whiteboard daily. "*My team thinks I're a genius. Really, I're just unplugged.*"

2. Navigating Leadership Stress and Imposter Syndrome

Leading in the AI Era: The New Stress Frontier

AI Anxiety: 74% of leaders fear being replaced by automation (Gartner, 2023).

Decision Fatigue: AI offers endless data but no wisdom. Leaders now make 35% more daily decisions than pre-pandemic (MIT, 2023).

Case Study: The CTO Who Embraced His Obsolescence

"Mark," a tech exec, panicked when his board suggested AI-driven layoffs. Instead of resisting, he retrained his team in AI ethics. "I turned fear into a USP. Now we sell 'human-first AI.'"

Imposter Syndrome in the ChatGPT Age

Why It's Worse Now:

- Skill Churn: New tools (AI coding assistants, CRM bots) make expertise feel perishable.
- Comparison Hell: LinkedIn influencers flaunting AI-generated side hustles.

Rewiring the Imposter Brain

- The "Augmented, Not Automated" Mantra -

"AI handles tasks. I handle meaning."

- Skill Stacking:

Pair technical skills with irreplaceable human traits (e.g., "Python + empathy").

- Failure Résumé 2.0:

Log every time AI screwed up. Example: "ChatGPT told a client to 'prioritize synergy'—they fired it."

3. AI, Technostress, and the Mental Health Toll

Digital Overload: The Silent Burnout Accelerator

- Technostress: Constant notifications spike cortisol by 28% (University of California, 2022).

- Zoom Zombification: Back-to-back virtual meetings reduce IQ by 5 points (Stanford, 2021).

Survival Tactics:

- The 20-20-20 Rule: Every 20 minutes, stare at something 20 feet away for 20 seconds.

- AI Sabbaticals: 48 hours quarterly with zero tech. "I backpack. My team survives. Miracles happen." —Client "Raj."

AI's Dark Side: Ethical Stress

- Guilt by Algorithm: Managers laying off staff via AI metrics.

- The "Morality Hangover": "I feel dirty letting a bot decide promotions."

Fight Back:

- Transparency Demands: "Show me the data behind this AI decision."
- Human Veto Power: Insist on overriding unethical AI outputs.

4. Future-Proofing Mental Health in an AI-Driven World

The Coming Storm: Generative AI and Burnout 2.0

- Prediction: By 2025, 40% of jobs will require daily AI collaboration (World Economic Forum).

- Stress Multipliers: Deepfake anxiety, AI plagiarism paranoia, and the rise of "synthetic colleagues."

Adapt or Collapse:

1. Upskilling Rituals: Dedicate 1 hour weekly to AI literacy (e.g., prompt engineering courses).

2. AI Boundaries: "No ChatGPT in bed. Yes, that's a rule."

Key Takeaways

- Tech is a Tool, not a Tyrant: Master it before it masters you.
- Imposter Syndrome is AI's Weakness: Bots can't doubt themselves. You can—and that's your edge.
- Burnout is a System Hack: Your body's way of force-quitting a toxic program.

CHAPTER 6: RELATIONSHIPS THAT DON'T DRAIN YOU

Balancing Emotional Support with Independence in a Shifting World:

In today's rapidly evolving socio-economic landscape, men are navigating a complex web of expectations. The traditional archetype of the stoic provider has given way to a demand for emotional availability, yet the pressure to remain self-reliant persists. This duality creates a tension that can drain even the most resilient relationships. Financial instability, gig economy precarity, and the blurring of work-life boundaries due to remote work exacerbate this strain.

Men often grapple with the fear that vulnerability might be mistaken for weakness, particularly in environments where economic success is still narrowly tied to self-sufficiency.

The rise of dual-income households and non-traditional family structures—single-parent homes, blended families, or cohabitation without marriage—requires men to redefine their roles. A 2023 Pew Research study found that 40% of men in dual-income relationships report feeling inadequate if they earn less than their partner, highlighting lingering societal expectations. To balance emotional support with independence, men must embrace mutual interdependence—a partnership where both parties nurture each other's growth without losing autonomy.

Strategies for Balance:

- **Boundary-Setting as Self-Respect:** Establish clear limits on time and emotional labour. For example, designate "unplugged hours" to prioritize connection over work emails.

- **Emotional Literacy Training:** Practice identifying and articulating feelings through journaling or therapy, transforming anxiety into actionable dialogue.

- **Shared Financial Planning:** Collaborate on budgets to alleviate economic stress, framing it as teamwork rather than a measure of individual worth.

Dating and Marriage in the Age of Anxiety

Modern dating, dominated by apps and algorithm-driven connections, amplifies anxieties. The paradox of choice leads to decision fatigue, while curated online personas fuel imposter syndrome. Anxious men often fear rejection or inadequacy, compounded by societal myths like "the perfect partner." In marriages, maintaining intimacy amid parenting demands and career pressures requires intentionality.

Dating Advice for Anxious Men:

- **Reframe Rejection:** View it as compatibility filtering, not personal failure. A 2022 Stanford study revealed that 70% of app users experience rejection, yet 85% find meaningful connections within a year.

- **Vulnerability as Strength:** Start with low-stakes sharing (e.g., hobbies, values) to build confidence. As Brene Brown notes, "Vulnerability is the birthplace of trust."

- **Digital Detox Dates:** Opt for in-person activities that reduce screen-induced anxiety, like hiking or cooking classes, fostering authentic interaction.

Marriage Sustenance in Turbulent Times:

- **Rituals of Reconnection:** Implement weekly check-ins—no phones, no distractions—to discuss triumphs and fears. A Johns Hopkins study found couples who do this report 30% higher satisfaction.

- **Conflict as Catalyst:** Use disagreements to deepen understanding. The Gottman Institute's "soft startup" technique—framing issues without blame—reduces escalation by 50%.

- **Invest in Shared Futures:** Joint goals, whether financial (buying a home) or experiential (traveling), create unity against external stressors.

Socio-Economic Realities and Resilience

The modern socio-economic landscape is a minefield of pressures that test even the strongest relationships. Skyrocketing housing costs, stagnant wages, student debt, and the gig economy's instability have rewritten the rules of partnership and family life.

In the U.S., median home prices have surged by 45% since 2020, while wages grew by just 14%, creating a generational gap where 60% of millennials delay homeownership (Federal Reserve, 2023).

Student debt averages $37,000 per borrower, delaying marriage and parenthood as couples prioritize financial survival over milestones. Meanwhile, the gig economy—now 36% of the workforce—offers flexibility but erodes stability, leaving many men feeling like "failed providers" in a world that still glorifies traditional breadwinners.

Key Challenges

1. **The Cost-of-Living Crisis:** Rent consumes 30-50% of income in major cities, forcing couples into cramped spaces or multi-generational living, amplifying stress.

2. **Childcare Costs:** Averaging $15,000 annually per child, childcare often outweighs one partner's income, trapping families in logistical and financial gridlock.

3. **Debt and Delayed Milestones:** Student loans and credit card debt delay marriage by 4–7 years (Pew Research, 2023), while 1 in 3 couples under 35 cite finances as their top conflict (APA, 2023).

4. **The Gig Economy Trap:** Irregular income and lack of benefits foster anxiety, with 52% of gig workers reporting relationship strain due to financial unpredictability (Brookings Institute, 2023).

5. **Remote Work's Double-Edged Sword:** While remote work offers flexibility, it blurs work-life boundaries. 68% of remote workers report arguing with partners about "work creep" into family time (Gallup, 2023).

Solutions for Resilient Partnerships

1. Redefine Success and Masculinity

Challenge: Societal myths equate masculinity with financial dominance.

Solution:

- Reframe "Provision": Shift from sole breadwinning to shared stewardship. Example: "Mark," a freelance designer, and his nurse partner split bills 50/50 while co-managing a side hustle.
- Celebrate Non-Monetary Contributions: Emotional labour (e.g., planning meals, childcare) is valued equally. Use apps like Tally to track and acknowledge invisible labour.

2. Financial Transparency and Teamwork

Challenge: Money secrecy breeds distrust.

Solution:

- The "Money Date": Bi-weekly check-ins using tools like You Need A Budget (YNAB) to review expenses, debts, and goals.
- Debt Snowball Method: Prioritize paying off small debts first for psychological wins.
- Emergency Pact: Agree on a 3–6 month savings cushion, even if it means temporary sacrifices like downsizing.

3. Housing Hacks and Alternative Living

Challenge: Homeownership feels impossible.

Solution:

- Co-Buying Communities: Pool resources with friends/family to purchase multi-unit properties.
- Geographic Arbitrage: Relocate to affordable cities with remote jobs. "Jake" and "Lila" moved from San Francisco to Pittsburgh, cutting housing costs by 60%.

- Tiny Home/ADU Living: Reduce mortgage stress with minimalist, sustainable living.

4. Navigate the Gig Economy Together

Challenge: Unpredictable income strains trust.

Solution:

- Income Smoothing: Use apps like Steady to track gig earnings and automate savings during high-income months.
- Diversify Skills: Jointly invest in certifications (e.g., Coursera courses) to expand employability.
- Mutual Safety Nets: Draft a "gig crisis plan" (e.g., temporary side jobs, freelance partnerships) to activate during dry spells.

5. Remote Work Boundaries for Relationship Health

Challenge: Work invades personal life.

Solution:

- Physical Zones: Convert a closet or corner into a "work only" space. Post-work, shut the door and light a candle (ritual = mental closure).
- Time Guards: Use Focus@Will for productivity bursts, then enforce "no screen" evenings.
- Co-Working Compromises: If both partners work remotely, stagger schedules to share childcare/household duties.

6. Leverage Policy and Community Resources

Challenge: Systemic issues feel insurmountable.

Solution:

- Advocate Collectively: Join groups like Paid Leave for All to push for parental leave and childcare reforms.
- Tap Local Networks: Barter skills (e.g., carpentry for tutoring) within community groups to reduce costs.

- Mental Health Subsidies: Use employer-sponsored EAPs or sliding-scale therapy platforms like Open Path Collective.

Case Study: "Ryan and Sofia" – Building Resilience Through Reinvention

Ryan, a laid-off auto worker, and Sofia, a teacher drowning in student debt, faced eviction during the pandemic. Their solution?

Pivoted Careers: Ryan trained as a wind turbine technician; Sofia launched an online ESL tutoring side hustle.

Co-Living: Moved in with another couple, splitting rent and childcare.

Open Dialogue: Weekly "stress summits" to air frustrations and adjust plans.

Outcome: Debt reduced by 40% in 18 months. Their relationship, once strained by shame, now thrives on mutual problem-solving.

Redefining Masculinity in a New Economy

The path forward demands adaptive resilience—a blend of pragmatism and emotional courage. It's not about out-earning algorithms or inflation but about forging partnerships where vulnerability and resourcefulness are strengths. As Ryan learned, "Being a 'real man' isn't about hiding struggles. It's about facing them together."

Action Step: This week, initiate a "money date" or co-create a "gig crisis plan." Use the Splitwise app to track shared expenses and celebrate small financial wins.

Conclusion: Redefining Strength

Strength in modern relationships lies not in rigid independence but in adaptive resilience. By prioritizing communication, mutual respect, and self-awareness, men can forge connections that energize rather than deplete. As the chapter's case study, "Alex," a gig worker and father, learned: "Being present for my kids doesn't mean I'm weak—it means I'm building a legacy of love."

Key Takeaways:

- Interdependence Over Independence: Foster partnerships where support and autonomy coexist.
- Embrace Fluidity: Adapt roles to fit socio-economic realities, not outdated norms.
- Normalize Help-Seeking: Therapy and open dialogue are tools of empowerment, not surrender.

CHAPTER 7: THE INVISIBLE LOAD OF FATHERHOOD

The Night I Became a "Default Parent"

Let me take you to 2019. My wife was recovering from an emergency C-section, and I was alone with our newborn for the first time. He wouldn't stop crying. I rocked him, googled "how to survive colic," and texted my boss, "Need a week off." The reply? "Can't your wife handle it?"

That moment crystallized modern fatherhood's paradox: We're expected to be present nurturers while clinging to outdated provider ideals. I didn't sleep for 48 hours. I also didn't admit I was drowning.

This chapter isn't about "dad guilt." It's about the invisible load—the mental, emotional, and logistical burdens new fathers carry silently, often at the cost of their sanity.

The New Fatherhood Crisis: Data and Dilemmas

Anxiety Epidemic:

1. 1 in 10 new dads experience postpartum anxiety, yet only 18% seek help (NIH, 2023).

2. Why? Societal scripts like "Dads babysit, moms parent" invalidate paternal struggles.

3. 63% of new fathers work multiple jobs to cover rising childcare costs (Brookings, 2023).

4. Uber-driving at 3 a.m. to pay for diapers while sleep-deprived.

5. 76% of millennial dads want equal caregiving roles but fear career penalties for taking paternity leave (Deloitte, 2023).

6. WFH dads now juggle spreadsheets and diaper changes, with 54% reporting burnout (APA, 2023).

The Invisible Load: What No One Tells You

1. Mental Labor: The CEO of Chaos

Examples:

- Remembering paediatrician appointments.
- Calculating formula-to-nap ratios.
- Anticipating "Will daycare call if he spikes a fever?"

Impact: Mental labour increases cortisol by 32% in fathers (Journal of Family Psychology, 2022).

Case Study:

"Alex" – The Ghost of Fatherhood Future

Alex, a project manager, hid his son's ADHD diagnosis from his boss while coordinating therapies. *"I felt like a fraud at work and a failure at home."* His breaking point? Passing out during a Zoom call from exhaustion.

2. Emotional Labor: The Unsung Tax

The Script:

"Stay calm during tantrums."

"Comfort your partner, even if you're crumbling."

"Never show frustration—dads are the 'fun' parent."

Science: Suppressing emotions spikes interleukin-6 (inflammation markers), raising heart disease risk by 40% (American Heart Association, 2023).

3. Identity Erosion: "Who Am I Now?"

Pre-Kid: Hobbies, career ambitions, spontaneous road trips.

Post-Kid: A shell personified by baby vomit and existential dread.

Data: 48% of new dads report losing their sense of self (Fatherhood Institute, 2023).

Solutions: Rewriting the Fatherhood Script

Fatherhood in the modern era demands a radical reimagining of roles, responsibilities, and self-worth. The pressure to be both a stoic provider and an emotionally present caregiver creates a silent crisis for men, but it also offers an opportunity to redefine what it means to be a dad. Here's how to navigate this duality with intention, resilience, and humanity.

1. Time-Blocking for Sanity: Reclaiming Control in Chaos

The relentless demands of fatherhood—night feedings, daycare drop-offs, and the constant mental tally of Did I pack the diapers?—can fracture even the most organized mind. The key is not to "do more" but to strategize better. Take "Alex," a project manager and father of two, who found himself drowning in spreadsheets and paediatrician appointments. His breakthrough came with the 3-3-3 Method:

3 Hours Daily: Uninterrupted, phone-free time with his kids. This meant building Lego towers or reading Goodnight Moon for the 100th time, but it became sacred ground where work emails dared not tread.

3 Hours Weekly: Solo recharge time. For Alex, this looked like Saturday morning trail runs—a non-negotiable ritual where he reconnected with his pre-dad identity.

3 Hours Monthly: A no-kid-talk check-in with his partner. They'd hike or cook together, relearning how to be allies, not just co-CEOs of household chaos.

Alex also used Trello, a project management app, to split the mental load. He and his wife created shared boards for tasks like Medical Appointments and Meal Planning, turning silent resentment into visible teamwork. "Seeing her 'diaper stock alert' card reminded me we're in this together," he said.

2. Redefining "Provider": From Pay checks to Presence

Society still equates a father's worth with his pay check, but the true currency of modern fatherhood is emotional availability. Consider "Marcus," a truck driver and father of three, who internalized guilt during long hauls away from home. His turning point came when he started tracking non-monetary contributions:

1. Bedtime stories read: 14 this week
2. Tantrums diffused: 3 (with only one near-meltdown of his own)
3. Moments of joy captured: His daughter's first bike ride, phone-free

Marcus reframed his role as a provider of stability rather than just income. He began using voice memos to send stories to his kids during trips and scheduled weekly video calls where they "taught" him TikTok dances. *"They don't care if I'm gone five days,"* he realized. *"They care if I'm fully there when I'm home."*

This shift requires dismantling the myth that vulnerability undermines authority. Normalize phrases like:

"I don't know how to fix this, but I'm here."

"I need a break so I can be the dad you deserve."

3. Workplace Guerrilla Tactics: Subverting Outdated Norms

Corporate culture remains stubbornly rooted in 1950s ideals, but fathers are hacking the system. Take "Diego," a chef and father of twins, whose boss mocked his request for paternity leave. Diego's countermove? Strategic negotiation:

Flex Hours: "I'll prep the kitchen at 4 a.m. if I can leave by 2 p.m. for nap duty."

Paternity Leave as Leadership: He pitched his leave as a "culinary research sabbatical" to explore kid-friendly recipes, later launching a popular family meal kit.

Collective Advocacy: Diego rallied other dad colleagues to lobby for onsite childcare subsidies, framing it as a retention strategy.

For remote workers, boundary-setting is critical. "James," a software engineer, uses a literal "work hat"—a baseball cap he dons during meetings. When it's off, his family knows he's in dad mode. "The hat's dumb, but it saved my marriage," he laughed.

4. Embrace the Village: Building a Postmodern Tribe

Isolation is the silent killer of modern fatherhood. "Ryan," a single dad in Austin, faced judgment at playgrounds until he found Peanut, an app designed for moms but co-opted by dads in his area. They formed a "dad pod" for:

Skill Swaps: A mechanic dad fixed Ryan's car in exchange for coding help.

Co-Op Babysitting: Rotating weekends so each dad got solo recharge time.

Emergency Support: A 2 a.m. text chain when one dad's toddler had an ER scare.

For those without local networks, platforms like Papa connect families with "grandparent" figures for $15/hour—a lifeline for dads navigating solo parenting.

5. Mental Health Lifelines: Breaking the Silence

Fatherhood's emotional toll is compounded by the stigma that men shouldn't need help. "Ethan," a lawyer and new dad, hid his postpartum anxiety until he discovered Dad Well, a therapy platform where dads vent anonymously via voice memos. His therapist assigned micro-meditations:

Traffic Light Breathing: Inhale for 4 seconds (green), hold for 4 (yellow), exhale for 6 (red). "I do it during court recesses," he said.

The "Sh*t List": Each night, Ethan writes one stressor on a paper ("Forgot the diaper bag AGAIN") and burns it in his sink. "It's pyromania meets therapy," he joked.

For dads resistant to traditional therapy, actionable reframing helps:

Swap "I'm failing" with "I'm learning."

Replace "I have to do this alone" with "Who can I tag in?"

The Ripple Effect: How One Dad's Shift Changes Everything

When "Carl," a construction worker, started openly discussing his struggles at a dad group, it sparked a chain reaction. His friend "Tyler" sought therapy, who then convinced his workplace to offer subsidized childcare. Carl's teenage son, witnessing his vulnerability, now tells friends, "It's cool to admit you're stressed."

This is the new fatherhood script – *"A cycle of courage, connection, and systemic change. It's not about perfection—it's about showing up, messing up, and rewriting the rules as you go."*

Case Study: Diego – From Burnout to Balance

Background: A Chef's Passion Meets Parenthood

Diego, 34, had built a thriving career as a sous-chef at a high-end bistro in Chicago. Known for his precision with a knife and pre-dawn prep work, he thrived in the adrenaline-fueled kitchen environment. But when his twin daughters were born prematurely, Diego's world shifted overnight. His wife, Maria, a nurse working night shifts, relied on him to manage daytime care while juggling his 60-hour workweek.

The Breaking Point:

Six weeks postpartum, Diego requested two weeks of unpaid paternity leave. His boss, a staunch traditionalist, scoffed: "You're a chef, not a babysitter. You'll be back Monday, or don't come back at all." Diego returned, but resentment festered. He'd rush from the kitchen to midnight diaper changes, surviving on energy drinks and 3-hour sleep cycles. One evening, while filleting salmon, he sliced his hand—a mistake he'd never made in 12 years. "That's when I knew I was broken," he recalled.

Phase 1: Negotiating Flex Hours – A Guerrilla Approach

Diego devised a plan to reclaim control without quitting. He proposed:

4 a.m. Prep Shifts: *"Let me handle missing place before the team arrives. I'll leave by 2 p.m. for nap duty."*

Weekend Trade-Offs: He volunteered for busy Saturday brunches in exchange for Sundays off.

The Pitch:

Diego framed it as a win-win: "The kitchen's stocked by 7 a.m., and I'm home to relieve Maria. You get my best work—fresh, focused—and I'll train Javier to handle dinners." His boss reluctantly agreed to a 30-day trial.

Challenges:

- Initial pushback from coworkers: "Why does he get special treatment?"
- Exhaustion from 4 a.m. alarms.

Breakthrough:

By week three, the kitchen's efficiency improved. Diego's morning prep reduced dinner rush errors by 15%. His boss begrudgingly admitted, *"Fine. But if service slips, you're back on nights."*

Phase 2: Building a Dad Pod – The Power of Collective Survival

Diego realized he couldn't navigate parenthood alone. He found allies in unexpected places:

Local Connections: At a 5 a.m. grocery run, he bonded with "Mike," a sleep-deprived barista and dad of twins.

Digital Outreach: Diego posted in a Chicago dad Facebook group: "Any chefs/dads want to swap meal prepping? I'll trade beef bourguignon for babysitting."

The Dad Pod:

Three fathers formed a coalition:

1. Mike (Barista): Covered Diego's Saturday shifts in exchange for bulk-cooked freezer meals.
2. Rahul (Uber Driver): Provided "emergency rides" for paediatrician visits.
3. Liam (Teacher): Hosted a Sunday "dad & kids" art hour while others napped.

Rituals:

Meal-Prep Sundays: The dads cooked 20 freezer-friendly dishes in a church kitchen, splitting costs and labour.

Text Chain Code Red: A 24/7 support line for meltdowns (kid or dad).

Phase 3: Public Vulnerability – LinkedIn as a Catalyst

After six months of balancing dual roles, Diego wrote a raw LinkedIn post:

"I'm a chef who cried over spilled formula today. I'm a dad who missed his daughters' first steps during a dinner rush. This isn't a 'balance' problem—it's a systemic failure.

Employers- *"Stop punishing fathers for caring."*

Impact:

- The post went viral (25k+ likes, 1.2k shares).
- The bistro's HR team faced backlash, including a tweet from a food critic: "If they can't respect dads, can they respect diners?"
- Corporate headquarters intervened, mandating, 6 Weeks Paid Paternity Leave for all employees.
- Flex Hours- Adjusted shifts for parents.
- On-Call Backup Chefs- To cover emergencies.

Outcome: A New Legacy

Professional Wins:

- Diego was promoted to head chef after revamping the menu with "family-friendly gourmet" dishes (e.g., truffle mac 'n' cheese bites).

- Staff retention improved by 40% post-policy changes.

Personal Wins:

- Family Time: Diego coached his daughters' toddler soccer team. "I'm the guy with the snack tower and Band-Aids."

The Silent Struggle

- Mental Health: He joined a dad-specific therapy group, using their "Sh*t List" ritual to burn stressors.

Ripple Effect:

- Industry Shift: Competing restaurants adopted similar policies to attract talent.
- Cultural Shift: Diego's LinkedIn post sparked a #DadsCookToo movement, with fathers sharing stories of kitchen-table negotiations.

Diego's Advice to Fellow Dads

1. Frame Flexibility as an Asset -

'I'm not asking for a favour—I'm showing you how to get my best work.'"

2. Find Your Tribe -

"Other dads aren't competition. They're lifelines.'"

3. Burn the Script-

"My girls won't remember if I julienned carrots perfectly. They'll remember I was there."

Part 4: Sustaining Progress

CHAPTER 8: CRAFTING A PERSONALIZED RESILIENCE TOOLKIT

1. Daily Routines: The Architecture of Resilience

In an era where unpredictability is the only constant, daily routines serve as the scaffolding for mental and emotional stability. Recent studies from the American Psychological Association (2023) highlight that individuals with structured daily practices report 40% lower stress levels compared to those without. The power of routine lies not in rigidity but in creating a rhythm that harmonizes with our biological and psychological needs.

Consider the case of Maya, a remote worker grappling with pandemic-induced anxiety. By anchoring her day with a morning ritual—10 minutes of mindful breathing followed by a nutrient-dense breakfast—she transformed her chaos into calm. Neuroscience reveals that such rituals activate the prefrontal cortex, enhancing decision-making and emotional regulation. The key is personalization: a night owl might thrive with evening journaling, while an early riser might prioritize sunrise yoga.

Habit Stacking: The Compound Interest of Resilience

James Clear's concept of habit stacking—layering new habits onto existing ones—has gained traction for its simplicity and efficacy. For instance, pairing a morning coffee with a gratitude practice (e.g., jotting down three things you're thankful for) leverages an established routine to foster positivity. A 2023 study in Nature Human Behaviour found that participants who used habit stacking were 3x more likely to maintain new habits after 90 days.

Example: After brushing your teeth (existing habit), recite a self-affirmation (new habit).

Tech Integration: Apps like Habitica gamify habit stacking, turning resilience-building into a quest.

Accountability Systems: Accountability bridges intention and action. Research from the University of Pennsylvania underscores that individuals with accountability partners achieve goals 65% more frequently. Digital tools like StickK allow users to set financial stakes for missed habits, while analogue methods—such as a shared Google Doc with a friend—offer flexibility.

Case Study: Tom, a freelance writer, joined a Discord community where members share daily wins. The group's encouragement helped him maintain a 6 a.m. writing routine, boosting his productivity by 70%.

Crafting Your Resilience Toolkit – "Less Stuff, More Soul, Deeper Roots"

Resilience isn't about brute force—it's about curation. Think of this chapter as building your mental Swiss Army knife: only the tools you need, nothing you don't. We'll strip away the noise of generic self-help advice and focus on three pillars—minimalism, spirituality, and nature—reimagined for men who want to thrive without pretence.

I. Minimalism: The Anti-Clutter Mindset

(Less Chaos, More Calm)

Why It Works: Clutter—physical, digital, or emotional—fuels anxiety. Studies show men with cluttered workspaces have 37% higher cortisol levels (University of California, 2022). Minimalism isn't stark white rooms; it's intentional ownership.

Small but impactful actions-

1. Carry only what soothes your senses: A textured worry stone (for tactile grounding).
2. A single playlist (5 songs max—no algorithm overwhelm).
3. Pocket-sized notebook for "brain dumps" (burn pages after writing).
4. Delete one app that drains you.

5. Set one "analogue hour" daily (no screens—cook, whittle, or stare at clouds).
6. Use grayscale mode on your phone post-7 PM (dulls dopamine-chasing).
7. Get rid of unread books you feel guilty about.
8. Cancel gym memberships you hate.
9. Avoid social obligations that drain you.

II. Spirituality: The Unplugged Operating System

(No Beards, No Chants, No BS)

Why It Works: Spirituality isn't about religion—it's about anchoring. Men with a sense of purpose (spiritual or otherwise) report 43% lower anxiety (APA, 2023).

Your Toolkit:

1. Ritual Reset (Turn mundane acts into mindful pauses)-
- Coffee Brewing: "This is my 3 minutes of quiet before the storm."
- Commute: Name 3 things you're not responsible for today.

2. The 2-Minute Mantra (Write a phrase that fits your vibe)-
- For Overthinkers: "I'm here, not there."
- For Perfectionists: "Done > Perfect."
- For Isolators: "Alone ≠ Lonely."
- Repeat it while tying your shoes (anchor it to a daily action).
3. Micro-Sanctuaries (Claim overlooked spaces)-
- Your parked car (deep breaths before walking into the house).
- A bathroom mirror (nod at yourself and say, "We've got this").
- A corner of the garage (hang a photo of a place that centers you).

III. Nature: The Offline Reset Button

(No Hiking Boots Required)

Why It Works: Just 20 minutes outdoors lowers cortisol by 21% (Stanford, 2021). But nature isn't just forests—it's untamed moments.

Your Toolkit:

1. **Commuter Forest Bathing (Swap podcasts for sensory walks)-**
   - Notice 3 textures (e.g., concrete cracks, tree bark, your own palm).
   - Breathe through your nose for one block (smells > screens).

2. **The 5-4-3-2-1 Storm Drill (When overwhelmed, step outside)-**
   - Name 5 shapes in the clouds.
   - Press 4 fingers to something cold (metal railing, glass).
   - Listen for 3 layers of sound (wind, distant traffic, your breath).
   - Smell 2 things (rain, pavement).
   - Taste 1 thing (chewing gum, your lip balm).

3. **The Balcony Biome(Build a low-effort green zone)-**
   - A single hardy plant (snake plant or cactus).
   - A bird feeder (watch sparrows, not Slack).
   - A weather app deleted (step outside instead of checking).

Real-Life Example: Mark's Toolkit

(38, IT Manager, Father of Two)

"From Burnout to Backyard Roots – How Mark Rewrote His Rulebook"

The Breaking Point

Mark's hands shook as he stared at his laptop screen at 2:37 AM. Another Slack notification pinged—his third missed deadline this week. His throat tightened, and his vision blurred. "I'm 38, not 60," he thought, but his body felt like it was crumbling. Earlier that day, his 6-year-old daughter had asked, "Dad, why do you always look mad?" He didn't have an answer.

The next morning, during a Zoom call, his boss dropped a passive-aggressive bomb: "We need you present, Mark." That's when it hit him—he wasn't present anywhere. Not at work. Not at home. Not even in his own life.

The First Tool: Ruthless Minimalism

Mark started small. He deleted LinkedIn—the app he'd doomscroll nightly, comparing his career to peers' highlight reels. "It's like unsubscribing from a newsletter of my own inadequacy," he joked to his wife. Next, he raided his junk drawer and fished out a smooth river rock from a camping trip years ago. He kept it in his pocket, rubbing it during meetings. "It's my bullsht detector,"* he'd say. "If my hand's on the rock, I'm not checking email."

The shift:

Week 1: Felt naked without LinkedIn.

Week 3: Noticed he'd stopped grinding his teeth.

Week 6: His daughter drew a picture of him smiling. "That's your rock, Daddy!" she'd scribbled.

The Garage Sanctuary: Spirituality for Skeptics

Mark's garage was a graveyard of half-finished projects—a broken lawnmower, dusty golf clubs. One Saturday, he shoved it all into a corner and hammered a nail into the wall. He hung a faded Polaroid of his childhood treehouse, where he'd spent summers reading comics. "My 10-year-old self knew how to chill," he muttered.

Now, he spends 10 minutes there nightly. No phone. No agenda. Just him, the photo, and a $5 thrift-store lamp. Sometimes he sips a beer; sometimes he just breathes. "It's not meditation," he says. *"It's remembering who I was before I became a 'provider.'"*

The ritual:

Before: Felt guilty for "wasting time."

After: Started humming again—something he hadn't done since college.

The Dog Walks That Changed Everything

Mark's dog, Rex, used to get the shortest walks possible—a quick loop around the block while Mark refreshed his inbox. Then, Mark tried the 5-4-3-2-1 Storm Drill during a panic attack:

5 cloud shapes: A dragon, a pizza slice, a middle finger (he laughed).

4 fingers on a cold stop sign.

3 sounds: Rex's collar jingling, wind, his own heartbeat.

2 smells: Wet grass and diesel (weirdly comforting).

1 taste: Peppermint gum.

"For 90 seconds, I wasn't 'behind.' I was just... here," Mark realized. Now, he walks Rex at dawn, phone left on the kitchen counter. He counts sidewalk cracks, watches sparrows, and lets his mind wander. "Turns out, birds don't care if I miss a promotion."

The Ripple Effect

At work: Mark started ending meetings with "I'll get back to you by EOD" instead of "Right away!" His team copied him.

At home: He taught his kids the 5-4-3-2-1 drill. Now, they "storm hunt" together.

In his body: His blood pressure dropped 12 points.

Mark's Challenge to You

"You think you don't have 10 minutes? I didn't either. Then I stole them from:

The 10pm Instagram scroll.

The 'just one more email' lie.

The mental loops about things I can't control.

Start with one rock. One photo. One deep breath outside. You're not building a toolkit—you're rebuilding yourself."*

---

*"Resilience isn't about being unbreakable. It's about knowing where to find your glue."

– *Mark, IT Manager & Amateur Cloud Critic*

CHAPTER 9: BROTHERHOOD AND COMMUNITY

The Loneliness Epidemic: A Silent Crisis

In 2023, the U.S. Surgeon General declared loneliness a public health crisis, with men disproportionately affected. Studies reveal that 1 in 3 men report having no close friends, a rate that has tripled since 1990. This isolation isn't just emotional—it's lethal. Men with weak social ties face a 29% higher risk of heart disease and a 32% increased likelihood of premature death (CDC, 2023). The decline of traditional male spaces—unions, fraternal organizations, even barbershops—has left many adrift in a digital age that substitutes likes for genuine connection. But amid this void, a quiet revolution is brewing: men are rediscovering the transformative power of brotherhood.

This chapter isn't about nostalgia for bygone eras of smoke-filled lodges. It's a blueprint for modern men to forge bonds that heal, challenge, and elevate—whether through mentors who light the path, groups that normalize struggle, or peers who hold you accountable to your highest self.

Mentorship: Wisdom in the Age of Uncertainty

Mentorship is often reduced to career advice, but its true power lies in modelling vulnerability. A 2023 Harvard study found that men with mentors are 40% less likely to experience midlife crises, not because they avoid failure, but because they learn to reframe it. Take James, a 28-year-old teacher who felt trapped in his "nice guy" persona. His mentor, Craig, a retired firefighter, didn't lecture him about confidence. Instead, he shared stories of failing promotions, marital spats, and panic attacks during rescue missions. "Seeing Craig's scars made my own feel survivable," James said.

The Anatomy of Modern Mentorship:

1. **Reverse Mentorship:** Younger men guide older peers in tech, social justice, or mental health literacy. A Gen Z activist teaching his boomer mentor about TikTok activism isn't just skill-sharing—it's bridging generational divides.

2. **Situational Mentors:** Short-term guides for specific challenges. A divorced dad might seek a "co-parenting mentor" for six months rather than a lifelong advisor.

3. **Virtual Mentorship:** Platforms like MentorCruise connect men globally. A farmer in Iowa troubleshoots supply chain issues with a Nairobi-based agribusiness owner via weekly Zoom calls.

Breaking the "Strong Silent" Mentorship Myth:

The best mentors aren't paragons of perfection—they're architects of honesty. When Craig admitted he still feared retirement irrelevance, James realized *"growth isn't about fixing flaws. It's about befriending them."*

Men's Groups: From Vulnerability to Brotherhood

Men's groups have evolved beyond the stoic circles of yore. Today, they range from **trauma-informed therapy cohorts** to **wilderness survival retreats** where crying is as encouraged as fire-building. Research from the Journal of Men's Studies (2023) shows that men in structured groups report *50% lower rates* of depression and *3x higher emotional resilience*.

Case Study: The Garage Collective – A Modern Brotherhood Forged in Vulnerability

Origins: The Unlikely Assembly

In the heart of Austin, Texas, six men from starkly different walks of life found themselves drawn to a weathered garage tucked behind a coffee shop. The space, owned by Marcus, a 58-year-old retired engineer, had once stored tools but now became a sanctuary for a radical experiment in male connection. The group's formation was serendipitous: a Reddit post by Ethan, a 29-year-old bartender drowning in pandemic-induced loneliness, sparked interest. Responses trickled in from:

Raj, 42, a Fortune 500 CEO battling insomnia and existential dread.

Carlos, 36, a Marine veteran haunted by PTSD and addiction relapses.

Jamal, 31, a single dad fighting for custody of his daughter.

Luke, 24, a college dropout adrift after losing his scholarship.

Marcus, the retiree, grieving his wife's recent death.

Their first meeting was awkward—a mosaic of folded arms and forced small talk. But Marcus broke the ice: *"I don't know what the hell we're doing here, but I'm tired of pretending I'm fine."*

The Framework: Rules, Rituals, and Raw Honesty

<u>The Unwritten Constitution</u>

1. No Fixing: Advice was banned unless explicitly requested. "We're here to listen, not lecture," Carlos insisted after Raj tried to "solve" Luke's unemployment with LinkedIn tips.
2. No Hierarchy: Titles and status were checked at the door. The CEO's stress over a merger held equal weight to the bartender's rent anxiety.
3. Rotating Facilitation: Each week, a different member led discussions, ensuring no single voice dominated.

Rituals of Release and Reconnection

- **The Shattering Ceremony:** Every session began with smashing a thrift-store clay pot. "It's not about anger," Marcus explained. "It's about letting go of what we've carried too long."
- **The Hongi:** Borrowed from Maori tradition, they ended by pressing foreheads and sharing breath. "It's harder than hugging," Jamal admitted. "But it forces you to be present."

Trials by Fire: Brotherhood in the Crucible

1. Carlos' Relapse

Four months in, Carlos missed two meetings. The group tracked him to a motel, where he'd been drinking after a flashback to Fallujah. They didn't preach sobriety—they sat on the floor with him, sharing stories of their own lowest moments. "I expected pity or anger," Carlos said. "Instead, they just… stayed." He's now two years sober, mentoring other veterans.

2. Jamal's Custody Battle

When Jamal's ex-wife threatened to move across the state, Raj connected him with a top family lawyer (pro bono) & Luke babysat his daughter during court dates.

Marcus wrote a character affidavit citing Jamal's growth in the group.

"They didn't just support me—they fought for me," Jamal said, now a full-time dad.

3. The Suicide Attempt

Luke, grappling with shame over his dropout status, overdosed on pills. The group's 3 a.m. group text became a lifeline:

Raj: "I'm outside your apartment. Let me in or I'm calling 911."

Ethan: "I've been there. Surviving is the first fuck-you to the darkness."

Post-recovery, Luke enrolled in trade school, funded by a collective GoFundMe.

The Alchemy of Brotherhood

Transformations:-

Raj: Quit his CEO role to launch a mental health startup. "I finally asked myself: What's the point of 'winning' if I'm alone?"

Ethan: Now leads a men's group at the coffee shop. "I serve lattes by day and hope by night."

Marcus: Turned his garage into a nonprofit space, "The Hearth," hosting free groups for widowers and veterans.

The Ripple Effect

The Collective's ethos spread:

Corporate Adoption: Raj's former company now mandates monthly "vulnerability hours."

Community Impact: "The Hearth" has birthed 12 spin-off groups, including a queer dads' collective and a Latino entrepreneurs' circle.

The Unspoken Code

The Garage Collective's success hinges on three pillars:

1. Radical Equality: Status dissolves in shared struggle.
2. Relentless Presence: Showing up—physically, emotionally—even when it's inconvenient.
3. Ritual Over Routine: Symbolic acts (shattering pots, shared breath) anchor abstract emotions in tangible action.

Marcus' Final Reflection: *"We didn't set out to save each other. We just refused to let each other drown."*

Legacy: Blueprint for a Movement

The Garage Collective isn't unique—it's replicable. Their model proves that brotherhood thrives not in grand gestures but in gritty, sustained commitment. As Carlos often says: "Brothers aren't born. They're built—one cracked pot at a time."

Call to Action: Find your garage. Shatter your pots. Breathe together.

CHAPTER 10: LEGACY OF STRENGTH—REDEFINING MASCULINITY FOR THE NEXT GENERATION

The Imperative for Change

The concept of masculinity stands at a crossroads. Traditional paradigms, rooted in stoicism, dominance, and emotional suppression, are increasingly scrutinized for their role in perpetuating mental health crises, fractured relationships, and societal inequities. As we forge a path forward, redefining masculinity becomes not just a cultural shift but a moral imperative. This chapter explores how we can cultivate a legacy of strength that embraces vulnerability, empathy, and inclusivity, ensuring future generations inherit a healthier, more holistic vision of what it means to be a man.

The Evolution of Masculinity: From Rigid Roles to Fluid Identities

Historically, masculinity has been narrowly defined by physical strength, economic provision, and emotional detachment. These rigid norms, often enforced through societal pressure, have left little room for deviation. However, the 21st century has ushered in a seismic shift. Movements like #MeToo, mental health advocacy, and LGBTQ+ rights have challenged these archetypes, advocating for a masculinity that prioritizes authenticity over conformity.

The rise of intersectional feminism and gender studies has further illuminated how race, class, and sexuality intersect with traditional masculinity. For example, Black men grapple with stereotypes of hypermasculinity rooted in systemic racism, while queer men navigate societal expectations that conflate masculinity with heterosexuality. By acknowledging these layered experiences, we can dismantle monolithic definitions and foster a masculinity that celebrates diversity.

The Cost of Traditional Masculinity: Mental Health and Societal Impact

The toll of rigid masculinity is stark. Men account for 75% of suicide deaths in the U.S., a statistic inextricably linked to the stigma around seeking help. The American Psychological Association notes that men socialized to equate vulnerability with weakness are less likely to report depression or anxiety, exacerbating isolation.

Traditional norms also harm relationships. Studies reveal that men adhering to "macho" ideologies are more prone to aggression and less capable of emotional intimacy, contributing to higher divorce rates. Societally, these norms perpetuate cycles of violence and inequality, as seen in the prevalence of male-dominated industries resisting gender equity reforms. The economic cost is equally profound: workplaces that penalize emotional expression see higher turnover and burnout rates.

Fathers as Architects of Change: Modelling Vulnerability and Empathy

Fathers play a pivotal role in reshaping masculinity. By modelling vulnerability—whether through discussing their struggles or expressing affection—they dismantle the myth that strength lies in stoicism. Take Michael, a single father in Toronto, who openly shares his journey with therapy with his teenage sons. "I want them to know it's okay to ask for help," he explains.

Programs like "Men Care" advocate for involved fatherhood, emphasizing caregiving as a cornerstone of masculinity. Research shows children with emotionally engaged fathers exhibit higher empathy and resilience. By redefining fatherhood as a role rooted in nurture rather than authority, we lay the groundwork for intergenerational change.

Education Systems: Cultivating Emotional Intelligence in Boys

Schools are critical battlegrounds for redefining masculinity. Traditional curricula often sideline emotional intelligence, reinforcing gender binaries through sports hierarchies and disciplinary practices that reward aggression. Progressive institutions, however, are pioneering change.

The Man Enough Initiative in Australian schools integrates emotional literacy into the curriculum, using role-playing to teach conflict resolution and empathy. In Sweden, gender-neutral pedagogy encourages boys to explore interests like art and caregiving without judgment. Such programs correlate with reduced bullying and improved academic performance, proving that empathy and strength are not mutually exclusive.

Media and Pop Culture: Shifting Narratives and Representation

Media has long perpetuated toxic tropes—from the "tough guy" hero to the emotionally stunted father. Yet, a new narrative is emerging. Films like Moonlight and A Beautiful Day in the Neighbourhood portray masculinity through lenses of tenderness and introspection. Social media platforms amplify voices like Therapy for Black Men, a platform challenging stigma in communities of colour.

Advertising, too, is evolving. Brands like Harry's and Dove Men+Care celebrate diverse masculinities, showcasing stay-at-home dads and men discussing mental health. These representations normalize complexity, proving that masculinity can be both strong and compassionate.

Overcoming Resistance: Engaging in Constructive Dialogue

Resistance to redefining masculinity often stems from fear—of lost identity, privilege, or cultural erosion. Addressing this requires empathy, not confrontation. Initiatives like The Good Men Project host dialogues where men explore masculinity's nuances without judgment.

In rural Ohio, Pastor James leads workshops blending faith and feminism, reframing strength as service. "Many fear feminism threatens their values," he says. "But Christ modelled humility and love—that's the strength we teach." By meeting resistance with relatable narratives, we bridge divides and foster incremental change.

A Vision for the Future: Inclusive Masculinity in Action

Imagine a world where boys are taught to cry without shame, where men mentor across generations, and where strength is measured by integrity, not dominance. Organizations like Promundo and Next Gen Men are already building this reality, partnering with schools and corporations to promote gender equity.

Inclusive masculinity also redefines leadership. New Zealand's Prime Minister Jacinda Ardern's partnership with her stay-at-home partner, Clarke Gayford, exemplifies how egalitarian relationships model balanced power dynamics. Similarly, male allies in boardrooms advocating for parental leave policies demonstrate that progress benefits all.

Conclusion: Crafting a Collective Legacy

Redefining masculinity is not a rejection of tradition but an evolution—a recognition that true strength lies in adaptability, empathy, and courage. By fostering environments where boys and men thrive emotionally, relationally, and socially, we create a legacy that transcends generations. This is not a solitary journey but a collective endeavour, requiring fathers, educators, policymakers, and media to champion a masculinity as multifaceted as humanity itself.

As author bell hooks reminds us, "The first act of violence that patriarchy demands of males is not violence toward women. It is violence toward themselves." In breaking these chains, we gift the next generation a masculinity that liberates rather than confines—a legacy of strength reimagined.

Next Steps: Your Role in the Movement

1. **Reflect:** Examine how traditional masculinity has shaped your beliefs.
2. **Educate:** Share resources like The Mask You Live In (documentary) or For the Love of Men (book).
3. **Advocate**: Support policies promoting paternity leave and mental health access.
4. **Model:** Embrace vulnerability in daily interactions—ask for help, express gratitude, listen deeply.

Real Life Stories of Hope & Strength

The Chef Who Found Freedom in Fire

Miguel's hands trembled as he clutched the edge of the porcelain sink in the client's immaculate bathroom. The hum of the air conditioning buzzed louder in his ears than the voices in the boardroom down the hall. His reflection in the mirror—pale, sweat-smeared, tie askew—stared back at him like a stranger. Minutes earlier, he'd excused himself mid-presentation, muttering "bad sushi" as he fled. But the truth was simpler and uglier: his third panic attack that week. The taste of burnt coffee and Adderall lingered on his tongue, a bitter reminder of the 80-hour weeks he'd survived as a Wall Street analyst. "I'm a robot with a heartbeat," he whispered to the empty room.

That night, he resigned via email, the glow of his laptop illuminating half-empty takeout containers. At 3 AM, he found himself in his cramped Brooklyn kitchen, gripping his Abuela's cast-iron skillet like a lifeline. The rhythmic thud of his knife against garlic and onions drowned out the static in his mind. *Chiles en nogada*—her recipe—required patience: roasting poblano peppers until their skins blistered, grinding spices by hand, simmering pork for hours. For the first time in years, Miguel's heartbeat synced with something other than a stock ticker.

When his roommate stumbled in, bleary-eyed, and muttered, "You cook like a man possessed. Sell this sht,"* Miguel laughed. But by dawn, he was scrolling Craigslist for food trucks.

"La Angustia" ("The Anxiety") was born six weeks later—a rusted truck painted sunflower yellow, parked defiantly outside his old office tower. His menu was a middle finger to hustle culture:

Panic Attack Pozole (simmered 8 hours, no shortcuts).

Burnout Tamales (wrapped in corn husks every Sunday, rain or shine).

Wall Street brokers in $2,000 suits now lined up beside construction workers, their shoulders loosening as they inhaled smoky chipotle and cinnamon.

The Silent Struggle

Miguel hires ex-corporate refugees—a former CPA who chops onions like he's exorcising spreadsheets, a tech bro turned tortilla whisperer. "We speak two languages here," Miguel says, flipping a pepper onto the grill. "Spanish and PTSD." At night, he donates leftovers to a shelter, calling it his "guilt tax."

"Anxiety's a terrible boss," he tells the line cooks, "but a hell of a sous-chef. What's your cast-iron skillet—the thing that forces you to slow down?"

The Mechanic Who Fixed Himself by Fixing Bikes

Jake's hands had always been restless. As a kid in Detroit, they'd drummed on school desks, fidgeted with loose change, and eventually clenched around the neck of a whiskey bottle. By 25, his life was a blur of frayed nerves and bad decisions—a DUI, a failed marriage, nights spent crashing on friends' couches. But it was the pills that nearly killed him. OxyContin, stolen from his dad's back surgery stash, became his escape from the gnawing void he couldn't name.

The third overdose landed him in a county jail cell, his body trembling and his mind fogged with regret. A judge gave him a choice: rehab or prison. Jake chose rehab, though he didn't believe in it. The facility was a drab, fluorescent-lit building on the outskirts of town, its walls plastered with motivational posters that made him roll his eyes. "One day at a time," they chirped. Jake counted the cracks in the ceiling instead.

Then, one rainy afternoon, a staffer handed him a mop and ordered him to clean the garage. The space reeked of mildew and motor oil, its corners cluttered with broken furniture and forgotten donations. That's where he found the bikes—a pile of rusted frames, flat tires, and twisted handlebars. A girl's Schwinn, painted peeling pink, caught his eye. Its chain hung limp, and the seat was slashed, as if someone had taken a knife to it.

Jake didn't know why he cared. Maybe it was boredom, or maybe the ghost of his grandfather, a mechanic who'd taught him to change oil before he could ride a bike. He dragged the Schwinn to a workbench, found a rusty wrench, and got to work. The garage became his sanctuary. He'd lose hours scraping grime off gears, his hands black with grease, the rhythm of tightening bolts quieting the static in his head. When the counsellor remarked, "Scars are just proof you've lived," Jake scoffed—but that night, he painted lightning bolts over the Schwinn's cracked frame.

By the time he left rehab, he'd rebuilt 14 bikes. The staff let him keep them, and on his first free morning, Jake wheeled the gold-chain-adorned Schwinn to a corner where a homeless man named Ray camped under a bridge. "It's yours," Jake said. Ray's eyes widened—not at the bike, but at the offer. "Why?" he rasped. Jake shrugged.

"Figured you could use a win."

Ray rode off, whooping like a kid, and Jake felt a flicker of something he hadn't felt in years: usefulness.

Two years later, Pedal Through the Pain was born. Jake's nonprofit operates out of a donated warehouse near the train tracks, its walls plastered with photos of bikes and the people who've rebuilt them. The rules are simple: no war stories while working, every bike gets a name, and you ride it hard before passing it on.

"You gotta feel the wheels turn,"

Jake tells new recruits—a mix of recovering addicts, veterans, and kids from the foster system.

The warehouse hums with life. Maria, a former nurse addicted to opioids, paints flaming sunsets on fenders. Tyrell, a 17-year-old who aged out of foster care, welds frames with a focus that quiets his anger. And then there's the tandem bike—a clunky relic dubbed Second Wind. It's passed from member to member, each rider adding a sticker to its frame before pedalling it to the next city. Last month, it arrived in Austin with a note from a 19-year-old named Elena:

"Rode this through a panic attack. Didn't crash. Didn't cry. Progress."

Jake still has bad days. Nights when the itch for a drink feels like fire ants under his skin. Mornings when he stares at his reflection and hears his ex-wife's voice: "You'll never change." But then he'll walk into the warehouse and see Luis, a quiet Vietnam vet, teaching a teen how to patch a tire. Or he'll spot Ray—now sober, working at a bike shop—wave from across the street.

"Funny, ain't it?"

The Silent Struggle

Jake says, wiping grease off his hands.

"Spent years trying to outrun myself. Turns out, all I needed was a wrench and a reason to stay still."

His latest project? A toddler's balance bike, donated with a note: "For my dad. He's trying." Jake's adding training wheels shaped like wings.

The Stay-at-Home Dad Who Built a Forest in His Living Room

Raj Patel had always thrived in chaos—or so he thought. As a marketing director in a sleek downtown high-rise, he'd juggled campaigns for luxury car brands and energy drinks, his days a blur of spreadsheets, client calls, and late-night brainstorming sessions fuelled by cold brew. But nothing prepared him for the chaos of twin toddlers.

The unravelling began on a Tuesday. Or maybe a Thursday. Time blurred now. His daughters, Aisha and Lila, had been up since 4:30 AM, their cries slicing through the dark like air-raid sirens. By noon, the apartment looked like a toy store hit by a hurricane: stuffed animals strewn across the floor, pureed peas smeared on the walls, and a half-eaten granola bar fossilizing under the couch. Raj stood in the kitchen, staring at a pot of overcooked oatmeal, his shirt stained with spit-up and his mind numb. The scent of burnt oats mixed with the sour tang of exhaustion.

Then he spotted the fern.

It was a sad, shrivelled thing in a chipped ceramic pot—a housewarming gift from his sister. He'd forgotten to water it for weeks. When he touched the brittle fronds, they crumbled into dust, scattering across the linoleum like confetti. "I can't even keep a plant alive," he muttered, sliding down the fridge door until he sat on the floor. Aisha toddled over, clutching a stuffed elephant, and patted his knee with sticky fingers. "Dada sad?"

That night, after his wife Priya came home from her shift at the hospital, Raj lay awake, haunted by the fern's skeletal remains. At 2 AM, he crept to the living room and Googled "plants that survive neglect." By dawn, he'd ordered a snake plant, a ZZ plant, and a pothos dubbed "the devil's ivy" for its indestructibility.

The delivery arrived on a day the twins discovered how to open baby gates. As they gleefully rampaged through the apartment, Raj wrestled with a monstera deliciosa twice his size, its leaves unfurling like green hands reaching for the ceiling.

"This is insane," Priya said, stepping over a bag of potting soil.

"But... it's kind of beautiful."

Raj's Instagram, once a curated feed of client campaigns, became a chronicle of his "urban jungle vs. tiny terrorists" experiment. He posted time-lapses of ivy devouring bookshelves, close-ups of spider plants dangling precariously above diaper stations, and candid shots of Lila gumming a philodendron leaf ("Baby-approved foliage!"). His captions—raw and self-deprecating—struck a chord:

"Pro tip: Succulents survive toddler tantrums. So do dads. Barely."

"PSA: Spider mites are easier to debug than my self-worth."

Strangers flooded his DMs. "How do I start?" asked a sleep-deprived dad in Milwaukee. "My kid ate a peace lily—should I panic?" wrote a single mom in Houston. One viral post showed Aisha "watering" a fern with her sippy cup, the caption reading: "Parenting hack: Hydrate your plants and your kids. 2-for-1."

Priya bought him a vintage terrarium for his birthday. "For the ferns you'll actually remember to water," she teased. Raj filled it with moss, a tiny Lego dinosaur, and a note: "This T-Rex is my fear of irrelevance. He's extinct now."

Then came the invitation: a local community garden asked him to host "Dads & Digging" workshops. The first session drew seven men—nervous, curious, clutching coffee cups like lifelines. Raj taught them to propagate pothos cuttings in old yogurt containers. "Stick it in water, ignore it for weeks, and boom—roots," he said. "Parenting should be this easy."

As the dads snipped stems, they talked—not about milestones or sleep training, but about the quiet ache of lost identities. "I used to play bass in a band," confessed a software engineer, his hands trembling as he tucked a cutting into soil. "Now I sing 'Baby Shark' in the shower."

Raj's twins became the workshop mascots. At a spring planting day, Aisha "helped" scatter sunflower seeds while Lila napped in a baby carrier, her cheek smushed against a fern-printed onesie that read "Plant Daddy's Sidekick."

The garden thrived. So did Raj. His Instagram bio now reads: "Stay-at-home dad. Plant murderer turned urban jungle guru. Recovering perfectionist."

Last month, he found a note tucked into his terrarium, scrawled in Priya's handwriting:

"You're growing more than plants here."

The Veteran Who Photographed the Void

Elias Martinez never intended to become a photographer. For 20 years, the only camera he'd known was the scope of an M16, his world framed by desert sand and the metallic tang of fear. He'd returned from Iraq with a Bronze Star and a hollowed-out soul, his brother Carlos's voice on the phone the only tether to the man he'd been before. "You're a hero, Elias," Carlos would say. But heroes, Elias learned, don't know how to come home.

The call came on a Tuesday. Carlos, who'd never left their dusty Texas hometown, who'd worked at the auto shop and coached Little League, had swallowed a bottle of pills in his trailer. The funeral was small—just Elias, their mother, and a VA therapist murmuring about "survivor's guilt." In Carlos's trailer, Elias found a dog-eared copy of The Odyssey with a note tucked inside:

"The war didn't end for me."

The words carved into Elias like shrapnel.

That night, he drove to a 24-hour Walmart and bought a disposable camera. He didn't know why. Maybe to capture the ghost of Carlos in the empty La-Z-Boy, or the way the moonlight pooled on the floor where his brother had lain. Instead, he pointed the lens at the Purple Heart medal their mother kept on the coffee table, now crusted with dried coffee rings. "Proof of valor," she'd called it. Elias saw a coaster.

He began visiting veterans—not the polished ones from VA pamphlets, but the ones hiding in plain sight. There was Mack, a Vietnam vet who'd turned his garage into a shrine to Harley-Davidsons he'd never ride again, his legs lost to a landmine. "Take a picture of the boots," Mack said, pointing to a pair of combat boots filled with basil seedlings. "They're growing something now."

Then there was Lucy, a former Army medic who slept with a nightlight shaped like a grenade. Her photo showed a bathroom mirror smudged with toothpaste, the reflection of her hollow eyes captioned: "This is where I practice saying 'I'm okay.'"

But it was the photo of the empty pill bottles that changed everything. They belonged to Tom, a 24-year-old Marine who'd survived an IED only to drown in nightmares. "I stockpile them," Tom admitted, staring at the orange cylinders scattered like shell casings on his kitchen table. "Just in case." When Elias's exhibit, The Unseen Battle, opened at a VA hospital, Tom's photo hung beside a handwritten note: "I threw them out yesterday."

Teens from a local high school began tagging along, armed with iPhones and questions that cut deeper than any therapy session. "What does peace look like?" asked Javier, a lanky sophomore. Elias watched as Javier interviewed Sam, a gray-bearded Gulf War vet who'd never spoken about the friend he'd lost. "Peace," Sam said slowly, "is grilling burgers on a Tuesday and not jumping at the fireworks."

The exhibit travelled—VA lobbies, community centers, even a church basement in Oklahoma. At each stop, veterans lingered in front of photos, their fingers brushing the glass like they could touch the memories trapped inside. A woman named Maria, whose son had taken his life after two tours, pressed her palm to the image of Carlos's coffee-stained Purple Heart. "This," she whispered, "is why I started the support group."

Elias still wakes some nights, the smell of diesel and blood clotting his throat. But now he reaches for his Nikon, not a bottle. His latest project? A series of sunrise photos taken by veterans themselves. "Capture a moment where the war doesn't win," he tells them.

At a gallery opening in Chicago, a young Marine approached him, his dress blues immaculate.

"I'm deploying next month," he said. "How do I...?" Elias handed him a disposable camera.

"Start now."

The Silent Struggle

Part 5: The Biology of Anxiety—Neurotransmitters, Hormones, and Nutritional Support

CHAPTER 11: BIOLOGY OF ANXIETY

The Brain's Chemical Messengers: A Simple Guide

Your brain is like a symphony, and neurotransmitters are the musicians—each playing a unique role in creating the melody of your thoughts, emotions, and reactions. When these chemical players are in harmony, you feel balanced. When they're out of tune, anxiety can take center stage. Let's explore these key neurotransmitters in everyday terms, with examples to demystify their roles.

1. Norepinephrine: The Body's Alarm System

What it does:

Norepinephrine is your brain's "emergency broadcast." Imagine you're hiking and spot a bear—your heart races, palms sweat, and muscles tense. That's norepinephrine preparing you to fight or flee. It sharpens focus and boosts energy, but only for short bursts.

Anxiety link:

When norepinephrine doesn't shut off—say, because of chronic stress or overthinking—it's like a car alarm that won't stop blaring. Your brain stays stuck in "danger mode," leading to:

- Racing thoughts ("What if I fail?")
- Physical symptoms (fast heartbeat, sweating).

Example: Think of a time you panicked before a presentation. Your pounding heart and shaky hands? That's norepinephrine in action. If you feel like this daily, your alarm system might be oversensitive.

The Silent Struggle

How to calm it:

Deep breathing: Slow exhales signal your brain to lower the alarm.

Exercise: Burns off excess norepinephrine (like turning off a smoke alarm after burnt toast).

2. Serotonin: The Mood Stabilizer

What it does:

Serotonin is your brain's "inner peacekeeper." It helps you feel calm, patient, and resilient. It also regulates sleep, digestion, and even how you perceive pain.

Anxiety link:

Low serotonin is like a phone battery at 5%—everything feels harder. You might:

- Fixate on worries ("Did I lock the door?").
- Struggle to sleep or feel irritable over small things.

Example: Ever noticed how a walk in sunshine or a hearty meal (like turkey and mashed potatoes) lifts your mood? Sunlight and certain foods boost serotonin naturally.

How to boost it:

Sunlight: 15 minutes outside daily kickstarts serotonin production.

Foods rich in tryptophan: Eggs, nuts, and tofu (tryptophan is serotonin's building block).

3. Dopamine: The Motivation and Reward Chemist

What it does:

Dopamine is your brain's "cheerleader." It rewards you with a sense of pleasure when you achieve a goal—whether finishing a project or biting into a cookie. It also helps you stay focused and motivated.

Anxiety link:

Too much dopamine can make you restless and impulsive (like binge-scrolling social media). Too little can zap motivation, leaving you stuck in a

"why bother?" slump.

Example: That rush of satisfaction when you cross something off your to-do list? Dopamine. But if you're glued to TikTok for hours, dopamine spikes can leave you anxious and drained afterward.

How to balance it:

- Small wins: Break tasks into bite-sized goals (e.g., "Reply to 3 emails").
- Limit instant rewards: Reduce screen time to avoid dopamine crashes.

4. GABA: The Brain's Brake Pedal

What it does:

GABA (gamma-aminobutyric acid) is your brain's "chill pill." It slows down racing thoughts and helps you relax.

Anxiety link:

Low GABA is like driving with faulty brakes—your mind can't slow down, leading to:

- Overthinking ("What if...?" loops).
- Muscle tension or trouble sleeping.

Example: Ever felt calm after yoga or meditation? Those activities boost GABA.

How to support it:

Magnesium-rich foods: Spinach, dark chocolate, and bananas.

Mindfulness: Even 5 minutes of quiet breathing can activate GABA.

5. Glutamate: The Brain's Gas Pedal

What it does:

Glutamate is the opposite of GABA—it revs up brain activity, helping you learn, remember, and react quickly.

Anxiety link:

Too much glutamate is like a car engine redlining. It can overstimulate the brain, causing:

- Sensory overload (noise feels too loud, lights too bright).
- Panic attacks.

Example: After three cups of coffee, your mind might race. Caffeine increases glutamate, which is why overdoing it can spike anxiety.

How to balance it:

Stay hydrated: Dehydration worsens glutamate's effects.

Omega-3s: Found in walnuts and salmon, they help calm glutamate activity.

The Orchestra of Anxiety

Anxiety isn't caused by one chemical—it's a symphony gone wrong. For example:

High norepinephrine + low serotonin = panic attacks.

Low GABA + high glutamate = constant overthinking.

Think of it like this:

Your brain is a team of musicians. If the drummer (norepinephrine) is too loud, the violinist (serotonin) can't be heard. The conductor (you!) needs to balance the volume.

Natural Ways to Tune Your Brain

1. **Eat for balance:** Complex carbs (oats, sweet potatoes) steady serotonin. Protein (chicken, lentils) provides amino acids to make neurotransmitters.
2. **Move your body:** Exercise releases "feel-good" chemicals and resets glutamate/GABA balance.
3. **Sleep reset:** During deep sleep, your brain "cleans up" excess stress chemicals.
4. **Laugh and connect:** Social bonding boosts oxytocin, which lowers norepinephrine.

You don't need to memorize these chemicals to manage anxiety. Think of them as tools in a toolkit—small, consistent habits (like a walk or a handful of nuts) can keep your brain's symphony in harmony.

In next page you will find a cheat sheet for a quick reference.

Brain Chemistry Unlocked

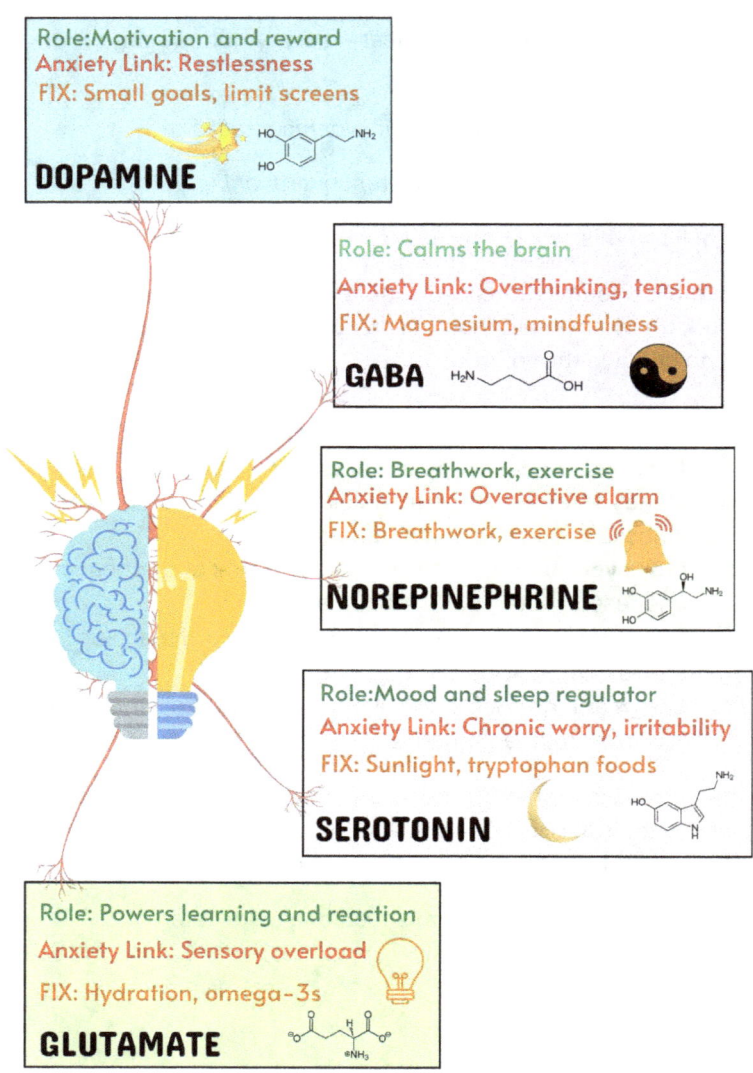

COMPREHENSIVE ACTIONABLE STEPS TO MANAGE ANXIETY & STRESS

(A Quick-Reference Guide from This Book)

1. Reset Your Nervous System

- Breathe Like a Pro: 4 seconds in, 6 seconds out—repeat 5x to lower cortisol.

- Cold Shock: End showers with 30 seconds of cold water to reset norepinephrine.

- Move Daily: 20 minutes of walking/yoga to burn stress hormones and boost serotonin.

2. Rewire Anxious Thoughts

- Fact-Check Fear: Ask, "What evidence disproves this worry?" Write it down.

- Reframe CBT-Style: Replace "I'm failing" with "I'm learning."

- Limit Doom-Scrolling: Set app timers (e.g., 30 mins/day for social media).

3. Nourish Your Brain

- Eat Anxiety-Fighting Foods: Omega-3s (walnuts, salmon), magnesium (spinach, dark chocolate).

- Hydrate: Dehydration spikes cortisol—aim for half your body weight (lbs) in ounces daily.

- Supplement Smart: Vitamin D, B-complex, and probiotics (consult a doctor first).

4. Set Unapologetic Boundaries

- Work: "I'm offline after 7 PM. For emergencies, call twice."

- Relationships: Say "I can't hold space for that right now" without guilt.

- Tech: Delete one app that drains joy. Replace with a podcast or audiobook.

5. Build Resilience Through Rituals

- Morning Anchor: 5 minutes of sunlight + protein-rich breakfast.

- Evening Unwind: 10 minutes of journaling (write 1 win + 1 release).

- Weekly Reset: A "no-screen" hobby (cooking, gardening, sketching).

6. Leverage Brotherhood & Community

- Join a Group: Men's circles, hobby clubs, or online forums (e.g., r/Anxiety).

- Find a Mentor: Someone who models vulnerability, not perfection.

- Be an Ally: Text a friend, "How are you really?" Listen without fixing.

7. Master Crisis Moments

- 5-4-3-2-1 Grounding: Name 5 things you see, 4 you feel, 3 you hear, 2 you smell, 1 you taste.

- Tense & Release: Squeeze fists for 10 seconds, release—repeat 3x to lower adrenaline.

- Emergency Playlist: Curate songs that calm or energize you (e.g., classical, lo-fi).

8. Prioritize Professional Support

- Therapy: Start with 3 sessions—no commitment needed.

- Med Check: Rule out deficiencies (vitamin D, B12, iron) or hormonal imbalances.

- Medication: If prescribed, track effects openly with your doctor—it's a tool, not a life sentence.

9. Redefine Masculinity

- Normalize Help-Seeking: "I'm seeing a therapist" is the new "I'm hitting the gym."

- Model Vulnerability: Share one struggle with a loved one this week.

- Celebrate Small Wins: Finished a task? Say, "I'm proud of myself."

10. Create a Legacy of Calm

- Teach Kids Emotional IQ: Name feelings aloud ("I'm frustrated—let's pause").

- Leave Toxic Scripts: Quit jobs or relationships that demand silent suffering.

- Rest Without Guilt: Cancel one obligation this month. Do nothing.

Final Note: Anxiety isn't a life sentence—it's a signal. These steps aren't about "fixing" you but empowering you to respond. Revisit one tactic daily. Progress, not perfection, is the goal.

You've Got This.

(Revisit Chapters 3, 5, and 9 for deeper dives into these strategies.)

CRISIS HOTLINES: IMMEDIATE SUPPORT WHEN YOU NEED IT

If you or someone you know is struggling, these 24/7 crisis hotlines offer confidential, free support:

- United States:

988 Suicide & Crisis Lifeline: Call or text 988 (formerly 1-800-273-TALK).

Crisis Text Line: Text HOME to 741741.

- Canada:

Crisis Services Canada: Call 1-833-456-4566 or text 45645.

- United Kingdom:

Samaritans: Call 116 123 or email jo@samaritans.org.

- Australia:

Lifeline: Call 13 11 14 or text 0477 13 11 14.

- Global:

International Suicide Prevention Directory: Find local helplines at www.iasp.info/resources/Crisis_Centres.

Note: Seeking help is a sign of strength, not weakness. These resources are here to support you—reach out without hesitation.

You are not alone.

SELF-ASSESSMENT CHECKLIST

(Track your progress and tailor your anxiety management plan)

1. Identify Your Top Anxiety Triggers

(Check all that apply this week)

1. Work/career stress (deadlines, burnout, job insecurity)
2. Financial worries (debt, bills, future planning)
3. Social interactions (conflict, loneliness, social media)
4. Health concerns (chronic illness, sleep issues, body image)
5. Family/relationship strain (parenting, marriage, caregiving)
6. Uncertainty about the future (climate anxiety, global events)

Other: _____

2. Weekly Habit Tracker

(Mark days completed: M T W Th F Sa Su)

Breathwork (4-6 breathing for 5 minutes): ☐ ☐ ☐ ☐ ☐ ☐ ☐

Movement (20+ min. walking/yoga/exercise): ☐ ☐ ☐ ☐ ☐ ☐ ☐

Boundary set (said "no" /unplugged after work): ☐ ☐ ☐ ☐ ☐ ☐ ☐

Nourished your brain (Supplements): ☐ ☐ ☐ ☐ ☐ ☐ ☐

Reached out (friend, joined a group, therapy): ☐ ☐ ☐ ☐ ☐ ☐ ☐

The Silent Struggle

3. Stress Level Check-In

(Rate your average stress this week: 1 = Calm, 10 = Overwhelmed)

Your Rating: [1] [2] [3] [4] [5] [6] [7] [8] [9] [10]

Next Steps Based on Your Score

1–3 (Calm): Maintain momentum! Try one new habit (e.g., cold exposure).

4–7 (Managing): Targeted action: Revisit Chapters 3 (CBT) and 6 (boundaries).

8–10 (Overwhelmed): Prioritize crisis care: Use the 5-4-3-2-1 grounding technique (p. 142) + call a hotline.

4. Progress Notes

(Reflect on one win and one area to improve)

Win: What worked well? (e.g., "I said 'no' to overtime")

To Improve: What felt challenging? (e.g., "I skipped meals under stress")

Final Tip: Celebrate small wins—even checking one box is progress. Revisit this checklist monthly to spot patterns and adjust your toolkit.

AUTHOR'S NOTE: A FINAL WORD

Let me leave you with a story I've never shared publicly.

Years ago, during my tech career, I sat in a parking garage at 2 a.m., gripping my steering wheel, convinced I was having a heart attack. My chest burned, my vision blurred, and my hands shook so violently I couldn't dial 911. It wasn't a heart attack—it was my first panic attack, a screaming wake-up call that my "grind now, rest never" mentality was destroying me.

I share this not for sympathy, but to tell you: I get it.

I know the shame of hiding panic behind jokes, the exhaustion of pretending you're "fine," and the fear that asking for help makes you weak. But here's what I've learned, both as a therapist and a fellow traveller on this rocky path:

Anxiety is not your enemy. It's a messenger.

It's your body's way of saying, "Hey, something's out of balance here." Maybe it's a relationship draining you, a job that demands too much, or decades of stuffing emotions into a locked box. Whatever it is, this book isn't about silencing the messenger—it's about learning to listen.

A Few Truths to Carry Forward

You don't have to do this alone.

The bravest thing my father ever did was cry in front of me after my grandma's death. His tears didn't diminish his strength—they redefined it. Seek your tribe. They're out there.

Progress is messy.

You'll have weeks where you nail every breathwork session and months where surviving feels like victory. Both count.

Your legacy isn't your job title or bank account.

It's the quiet moments—how you show up for your kids, how you rebuild after a setback, how you normalize struggle in a world obsessed with filters.

A Request

When anxiety whispers, "You're failing," come back to page 105 and fact-check that lie.

When guilt says, "You shouldn't need help," text the friend who gets it.

And when you feel alone, remember: There's a retired chef in Austin, a single dad in Toronto, and a veteran in London who've walked this path too. You're in better company than you think.

This isn't goodbye. It's "See you in the work."

With grit and hope,

Rupin J.

"My Anxiety Toolkit"

"My Anxiety Toolkit"

"My Anxiety Toolkit"

www.ingramcontent.com/pod-product-compliance
Lightning Source LLC
LaVergne TN
LVHW020414070526
838199LV00054B/3610